BOND

BOND

The 4 Cornerstones of a Lasting and Caring Relationship with Your Doctor

KEN REDCROSS, MD

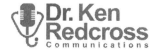

Published by
Dr. Ken Redcross Communications, Inc.
NEW ROCHELLE, NEW YORK
www.DrKenRedcross.com

The information and advice contained in this book are based upon the research and experiences of the author. They are not intended as a substitute for consulting with your physician or other healthcare provider. The publisher and author are not responsible for any adverse effects or consequences resulting from the use of any of the information or suggestions presented in this book. All matters pertaining to your physical health should be supervised by a healthcare professional who can provide medical care that is tailored to meet individual needs.

Editor: Carol Killman Rosenberg • www.carolkillmanrosenberg.com
Cover & interior design: Gary A. Rosenberg • www.garyarosenberg.com

ISBN-13: 978-0-69213-800-7

Printed in the United States of America

Contents

Forewords by Phylicia Rashad and Judge Greg Mathis.... ix

Preface..xiii

Introduction...1

1. The 4 Cornerstones of the Patient-Doctor Bond........7

2. Trust: Laying the First Cornerstone.................. 17

3. Communication: Exchanging Information
   for Mutual Benefit.................................. 37

4. Respect: Treating Each Other with Honor
   and Dignity....................................... 57

5. Empathy: Seeing Each Other from a Common
   Perspective....................................... 83

6. Time to Assess: Filling Out the Patient-Doctor
   Relationship Evaluation 101

7. A Conversation with Dr. Redcross: Common
   Patient Questions Answered....................... 113

Conclusion... 131

Author's Note to Fellow Doctors 133

Acknowledgments................................... 137

References... 139

About the Author 143

To all my patients, past and present:
May we always share an unbreakable bond.

Foreword

Healthcare is a personal matter. It is, therefore, reassuring to know that your healthcare is being supervised and administered by a well-trained, experienced medical professional with a personal investment in your physical health and overall wellbeing. I am referring to the patient-doctor relationship—a bond of mutual trust—that Dr. Ken Redcross elucidates in this book. This is the relationship that he would see brought back to the forefront of the healthcare system in our country today.

I grew up in a time when a doctor's visit to one's home was not unusual. In fact, it was quite normal. There was warmth and comfort associated with these visits that put the mind at ease and supported health and healing. With advancements in medical technology and growth in population, as well as in the healthcare industry itself, we have moved away from this method of care into one that is more impersonal.

Imagine, if you will, my chagrin some ten years ago, at meeting a young doctor whose interest lay in having the patient-doctor relationship be at the heart of his growing practice. I was stunned! I was equally delighted and impressed by his inquisitive nature in finding and studying alternative methods, treatments, and solutions to add to his storehouse of knowledge of traditional medicine- all for the benefit of his patients' health.

Having known Dr. Redcross and been on the receiving end of his knowledge has been most beneficial to me, as well as to friends and associates to whom he has been introduced. All have shared the same observations, the same sentiments: "This approach is very different. There is a real relationship here that makes such a difference. Thank you!"

In this volume, Dr. Ken Redcross shares his experience and understanding of the importance of the patient-doctor relationship for the benefit of patients and doctors alike. It is my hope that it will be of service to you as it has been of service to me and to others.

—Phylicia Rashad

Phylicia Rashad is an American actress, singer, and stage director. She is well known for her role as Clair Huxtable on the NBC sitcom The Cosby Show.

I first met Dr. Redcross more than a decade ago at a holiday party. We started talking, and the conversation somehow migrated toward healthcare and where we thought it was headed in this country. It was mutually understood that many people—too many people—were frustrated with their care. In speaking with Dr. Redcross, I learned that it wasn't just patients who were suffering emotionally; doctors were feeling overworked, underappreciated, and thoroughly discouraged. When I asked Dr. Redcross what he thought could solve this massive, complex problem, he had a simple answer: bringing patients and doctors closer together into a strong, healthy, lasting relationship. Put more simply: We should all be treating each other like family.

Growing up in Detroit with rather humble beginnings, love of family had always been the most important thing in the world to me, and it still is to this day. Your family—whether the one you're born into or the one you choose—is the rock that you can build your dreams upon. It's the support system that gets you on your feet—and helps keep you there. These are the people who will care about you unconditionally—will never judge, will never demean, will only love.

Imagine having a physician who feels like that, like a member of your family. I found it to be quite a forward-thinking concept when Dr. Redcross first introduced it to me, but it makes so much sense. You're trusting your doctor with one of the most valuable things you possess: your health. You're having to open up and divulge things that you'd never tell a stranger. You're exposing yourself—your body, your thoughts, your fears. You're asking someone to listen to you, really hear you, really understand you, really see you for all that you are: a human being.

This can't be about waiting rooms and appointment bookings and prescription pads. This can't be a cold, clinical, transactional relationship. This is so much bigger than all of that.

In working with Dr. Redcross as a patient of his concierge practice, we formed a close relationship that gave me some first-hand experience of the patient-doctor bond in action. Let me tell you, it's a powerful thing. No matter what city I was in, Dr. Redcross would be there. No matter how busy our schedules were, he would make me a priority. No matter what the clock read, he would give us all the time we needed. This relationship—built on trust, communication, respect, and empathy—not only improved my health and warmed my heart, but it transformed my perspective. It led to a wonderful epiphany: *This* is how healthcare should be—for all of us.

Looking at what's going on right now with healthcare in this country, it's clear to me that something is broken. No matter what side of the aisle you're on, you surely see it, too. There's financial hardship. There's oppression. There's an excess of political gamesmanship and a lack of human empathy. Now, there's a lot we need to do on the road to patching ourselves up. It'll take more than a few stitches. But every problem that was ever solved was solved by taking one step at a time. This is just one step, but it's one that we can all take, right now, together.

The relationship we have with our doctors can—and should —be a special one. Let's work at it. Let's tend to it. Let's cherish it. Let's not underestimate it. Let's never give up on it.

—Judge Greg Mathis

Judge Greg Mathis is a retired Michigan 36th District Court judge and syndicated television show arbiter on the long-running reality courtroom show Judge Mathis.

Preface

It is 2012, and I look out into an audience of 250 physicians staring back at me—all of them more experienced, many of them skeptical, some of them outright adversarial—and pitch my platform for delivering care at our practice. I take all of their disagreement and distrust, bottle it up, and magically transform it into strength, based solely on my firm belief that I have a higher purpose: I am here to support these doctors, increase healthcare efficiency, and improve the patient experience. I am here to *change the world*.

To the tune of polite applause, I leave the stage feeling confident and proud of a job well done. Honestly, I feel a little vindicated, too. The only problem? Other than that, I feel nothing.

After working in several medical groups on their leadership teams, I had explored the administrative world, starting in business school in the hopes of becoming a chief medical officer so that I could have a greater impact on doctors' lives and patient care. Before I even had the chance to graduate, the former CEO of a medical group approached me with the opportunity to run a relatively large medical group in the Tri-state area. It was a serious personal challenge, but one that I found exciting. True to form, I tackled it with full force.

The new job demanded a lot from me: long hours, a lengthy commute, impromptu meetings late in the day, and so on. And as a brand-new chief medical officer, without an MBA, the older, more seasoned doctors made it very clear to me that I had to earn my stripes. I could almost hear what they were thinking: *Who is this young guy coming in, telling us what to do?*

I didn't blame them. But I did try to sway them. And, as they got to know me, I began to win over many of these physicians and gained their critical support. Yet even though the job became easier and I had advocates, a nagging thought still lingered in my mind.

When it came time to stand before all those doctors in what was, until that point, the biggest moment of my career, it suddenly became too obvious to ignore: *Something was missing.*

So, following my presentation, I went to the chapel that I frequently visit during times of stress (which aren't few and far between), seeking peace. I took in the breathtaking view—a serene landscape the very picture of heaven—and began to pray.

"God," I said humbly, "I ask for clarity. I don't know what's going on. But I know that I'm missing something. Please help me understand."

Amidst all of my stress and anxiety, a new feeling arose. It was this hollow sensation above my gut and under my rib cage that was quickly followed by the greatest clarity I have ever experienced in my life. And then a voice spoke: "Change lives."

Look, I didn't grow up in the church. But I do believe in a higher power. And sitting there in that chapel, I could only describe it like this: It's as if someone was right there in the room with me, giving me direction, telling me my life's purpose. "Change lives." The clear and simple phrase filled my heart and saturated my soul. Instantly, all of the angst and uncertainty melted away. I saw the sun shining. I heard birds chirping. (Seriously!) And I was no longer afraid. In this world of 7 billion people, I now knew what I had been personally called to do.

Within two weeks, I quit my job—leaving the fancy title and high-paying salary behind—and went back to being a primary care doctor so that I could focus on what has always mattered most to me: the patient-doctor bond. I realized that during my time as a chief medical officer, I had missed that direct, spiritual connection with people. I was too far away from the human level to have a real impact on individual lives. I had been up at 30,000 feet. It was time to return to sea level.

I have recommitted myself to changing the lives of others by bringing love and happiness back to the patient-doctor relationship, and this book has sprung from that commitment. It is my hope that what was once a gap between patients and doctors will become a solid bond that leads to what I call "patient nirvana." In other words, I want patients to leave their doctors' offices feeling happier than when they went in. I want patients "floating" out of the room after an appointment because they feel like their questions have been answered, their fears have been addressed, and they don't have to worry because their doctor is on their side.

Is that possible? I know it is because that is what I aim for every time I see a patient. When we take a heart-centered approach to each other as human beings and remember that we are all made from the same mold, it doesn't have to be such an uphill challenge for us to be happy together. We can achieve health and healing as a team. It simply takes a sincere desire between a patient and doctor to build a lasting, caring bond.

Introduction

I can't tell you how many times I've heard people say, "My doctor doesn't listen to me. I feel like I'm not being understood," and physicians say, "My patients have no idea how much I deal with on a daily basis." It's true that today's doctors are facing longer hours and more jam-packed schedules than ever before, and they find it more and more difficult to give patients the time and attention they deserve. Meanwhile, patients are upset because their doctors don't have the time to hold a real conversation, aren't speaking in terms that someone who didn't go to medical school can understand, and are quick to just write a prescription. This makes for a lot of frustrated people on both sides of the stethoscope.

It's no surprise that healthcare happiness is becoming more and more elusive. Over the past few decades, the United States has been facing a sharp decline in primary care doctors. The Association of American Medical Colleges predicts that the country will be short between 14,900 and 35,600 primary care doctors by the year 2025.[1] This crisis is due to many factors, including a growing and aging population, millions of newly insured Americans, and declining interest in the primary care profession. In a recent study, only 2 percent of medical students had interest in practicing primary care, instead wanting to pursue specialty fields like dermatology or radiology.[2] And who can blame them? Family medicine physicians generally earn about half the average annual salary of specialists in dermatology, cardiology, and radiology.[3] Why would someone attend medical school for the same four years and pile on the same amount of debt (an average of $170,000) just to earn a portion of the same salary? Often, the reason primary care doctors make that less lucrative choice is because they love, like I do, spending a lot of one-on-one time with patients to form long-term, meaningful relationships. But what happens when stress, pressure, and unrealistic expectations start chiseling away at those relationships?

Due to the sharp decrease in primary care physicians and an influx of patients, doctors are often overscheduled. On average, a primary care doctor will see twenty to thirty patients a day, getting to see each patient an average of just seven-and-a-half minutes at a time. Medicine has become a mill, based more on volume than on value. And that's not why any of us went to medical school. We wanted to have a meaningful impact. We wanted to, well, *change lives.*

The patient-doctor bond is on faulty ground, and it has been for a while. We need to come together to heal the foundation that creates a strong patient-doctor bond. That's what this book is about. It's a place for all of us—patients and doctors—to literally get on the same page, listen to each other's fears, concerns, complaints, hopes, and dreams, and fully understand each other so that we can finally achieve a truly harmonious relationship that makes our lives better.

While I mostly address, you, the patient throughout this book, I have insightful information and advice to share with my fellow doctors, which you'll find at the end of every chapter.

But to truly understand one another, we need to consider both perspectives, so I encourage you to read the book straight through. I've also included features in the chapters called "Behind the Curtain" where I share with you some personal anecdotes from my career. In these sections, I hope to convey to you what it means to me to create a familial bond with the people who come to me seeking care.

I firmly believe that a doctor should feel like a member of a patient's family. That's the ultimate goal. Because when you feel like your doctor is part of your family, you can open up to them and talk freely without fear of being judged. This means that you'll be less likely to keep pertinent health information from them, which leads to faster diagnosis and treatment. You're also more likely to trust your doctor and follow their advice. In fact, research shows a strong correlation between the strength of the patient-doctor relationship and adherence to a doctor's recommendations.[4] Unfortunately, a high percentage of patients, according to a 2012 meta-analysis by Kevin Cheung, et al., do not follow their doctor's advice, which ultimately leads to a reduced quality of life and increased healthcare costs. While several contributing factors are likely at play, lacking the necessary level of trust in the patient-doctor relationship is a major one. How many lives could be improved if cultivating a strong patient-doctor bond is made a priority in healthcare?

Think about your relationship with your doctor. Do you take what your doctor says to heart and follow their recommendations? Do you feel like you can tell your doctor anything? Do you know with certainty that you can trust your doctor with your health? Do you believe that your doctor cares about you as a person? Should you even expect your answers to any of these questions to be yes? Of course you should—and it *is* possible to have this type of relationship with your doctor.

We all want to reach "patient nirvana," and this is your guide for how to get there. How many times have you asked someone, "Do you know a good doctor? I need a new one." I want you to never have to ask that question ever again. In this book, I'm going to lay it all out there and give you some insight into what a doctor deals with on a daily basis. For the most part, I want you to know that doctors are doing their best. Their whole goal is to make you healthy and, as a result, happy. But I'm also going to talk about how doctors might turn patients off and how they can change that if they are willing. I'll give you tools and tips to strengthen your relationship with your doctor and offer ideas on how your doctor might strengthen their relationship with you. But, most important, I'll outline the foundation of an ever-lasting patient-doctor bond. Yes, it takes extra effort on everyone's part to build this foundation, and we might have to dig down deep into the earth, but the result will be greater healthcare happiness for all.

I believe that true happiness is found when we consider that there is a deeper meaning to life than just getting by; we take that extra step, make the extra effort, and speak and act from our heart. That's why one of the things I often ask my patients is: "How's your soul?" And I ask that because I believe that at the very core of every relationship—including the one between patient and doctor—is a journey to find your soul, or spirit. It's about understanding your purpose in life, your impact on the lives of others, and your power to change your own. In a healthy, lasting patient-doctor relationship, this is a journey that never truly ends. But it has to start somehow. Come along on that journey with me. It starts now.

In chapter 1, I'll introduce you to the four cornerstone qualities that support a strong patient-doctor bond. These are the essential elements of any healthy relationship. Then, in chapters 2 through 5, we'll examine each of these qualities in depth to get a really good understanding of how to cultivate them and avoid the common pitfalls. In each of these chapters, I'll also share with you real-life examples of how my patients and I strive toward "patient nirvana" and conclude our patient-doctor experience with a sincere smile. I have no problems sharing with a patient some of my personal feelings, and I hope that provides a platform for them to understand that my office is a safe space, a "special zone" where we can both experience stability and comfort.

Each chapter closes with tips for cultivating the cornerstone qualities in your relationship with your doctor based on the information shared in the chapter. For my fellow doctors who are taking the time to read this book, I'll include a special feature called "From Doctor to Doctor" at the end of each chapter to share with you my take on how you can improve and strengthen your relationships with your patients based on my own experience and observations.

And since we're all in this together—all part of the same human network—both patients and doctors can gain a deeper understanding of the other by reading the parts of the book that don't specifically address them. I encourage you to do this to get a complete picture that can help us come to a mutual understanding for our collective healthcare well-being.

My advice is offered with pure intentions. If a doctor disagrees or feels they don't have time to implement my ideas, I respect that. It's important to keep in mind that we are all unique individuals—what works for one may not work for everyone. Therefore, I encourage both doctors and patients to take from my advice and ideas what works for them. Hopefully, in this way, we can find common ground.

Chapter 6 is an opportunity to assess your current patient-doctor relationship. If you find that you are dissatisfied with the relationship you have with your current doctor, you can use the information and tips in the book to start building a more mutually satisfying relationship. However, if you feel that you would be better served by a different doctor, you'll find some useful advice on that topic as well. In the final chapter, I offer my perspective on subjects that are the basis of many of the common questions I hear from my patients, and I hope this "one-on-one" time will provide you with some information on the topics you may be curious about and maybe want to bring up with your own doctor.

My honest hope for this book is that it helps you move closer toward "patient nirvana." We'll take it one idea, one cornerstone quality, at a time. Hopefully, by the time you close this book, you'll have a solid idea of how to create a lasting, caring bond with your doctor and can get started at your very next appointment.

CHAPTER 1

The 4 Cornerstones of the Patient-Doctor Bond

"We need people in our lives with whom we can be as open as possible. To have real conversations with people may seem like such a simple, obvious suggestion, but it involves courage and risk."

—THOMAS MOORE

People who stand by you through tough times, hold you up when you're not at your best, help you make important decisions, and share in your joy when everything is going well— that's what supportive family is. Supportive family members are there for one another and work together to achieve common goals. They care for and understand each other. They share a special, virtually unbreakable bond.

Isn't that also the role a doctor plays in your life . . . or should? When you're dealing with something as significant and intimate as your health, what better ally could you ask for than someone you think of as a close family member? Who better to look out for your best interests and help you make good choices when it comes to your health and well-being than someone you consider part of your inner circle? There's no one better, and that's why I firmly believe that the doctor you see should feel like a valued member of your family—and you a part of theirs. That's how I operate in my practice and what I aim to foster in my patients.

My goal is to help you learn how to build and maintain that type of patient-doctor relationship if you don't already have one. I want to help you figure out what might be missing from your current relationship with your doctor if you don't feel supported and what to look for in a new doctor if your new health plan gives you no choice but to find a new primary care physician. It all starts with understanding the building blocks of any healthy relationship.

Whether with family members or with your doctor, the cornerstone qualities that support a strong bond are the same: 1) Trust, 2) Communication, 3) Respect, and 4) Empathy. No one quality is more important than the others. Each one is essential in creating a balanced foundation that supports the bond. If one cornerstone is missing, eventually the whole structure collapses. What's more, without one of these cornerstones, a solid patient-doctor bond couldn't exist in the first place. And, remember, it's a two-way street. To truly create a lasting patient-doctor bond, effort and desire are necessary on both sides.

Trust

The first of the four cornerstone qualities is trust. *Trust* is defined as having confidence or faith in someone or something. However, trust between people isn't as cut and dried as a dictionary definition. Depending on the people involved and the

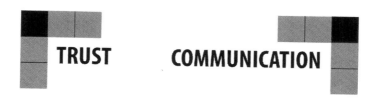

THE 4 CORNERSTONES OF
THE PATIENT-DOCTOR BOND

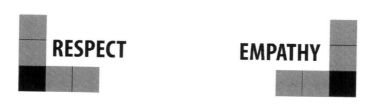

details of the situation, there are different levels and requirements of trust. In chapter 2, we'll get into the nuances of trust and how it is both forged and broken—with an emphasis, of course, on cultivating this important quality in the exam room. But, generally, it's enough to understand that, from the get-go, trust plays an essential role in the doctor-patient relationship.

When a patient visits their doctor, it's usually not because things are going well. More often than not, they're coming in to discuss a problem with their health, whether that's a chronic condition or a worrisome new development. And even if they're coming in for an annual checkup, there's likely still some level of anxiety, concern, or simply a fear of the unknown.

A person in need of healthcare visits a doctor with a certain level of trust going in. They trust that the doctor is in good standing with the medical board, will give them the care and attention required to accurately diagnose the problem, and will offer the best prescriptive advice they can with the information they have. Simply making the appointment indicates that this basic level of trust exists.

Then, during the visit, the patient is asked to share personal information about their health and their life in order for the doctor to reach the right diagnosis and treatment plan. This trust goes a little deeper. For a patient to open up, they need to trust that their doctor will listen, understand, respect their privacy, care for them, and won't judge or shame them. At the same time, the doctor needs to trust that their patients are being completely honest with them and will follow through with their recommendations to regain and/or maintain their health or let them know when something is not working for them.

The key to medicine is the back-and-forth sharing of information. And there can be no sharing without trust.

Communication

Communication is at the core of every human interaction. Without the ability to communicate, the world would be chaotic and, frankly, frightening. However, the ability to communicate doesn't necessarily mean that we are doing it well. Developing healthy communication habits takes practice, effort, and willingness.

Healthy communication is the tool by which any good relationship operates. It is comprised of several factors—clarity, authenticity, humility, and courage, among others. Without clear communication, patients and doctors run the risk of missing key pieces of information, leading to potential misdiagnoses or ineffective treatment recommendations on the doctor's part and misunderstandings regarding medical details and recommendations on the patient's part. I always want my patients to leave an appointment knowing as much as I do about their current state of health, which means speaking in terms they can understand and feel good about.

Just as important, two-way communication ensures that each party can come to understand where the other is coming from. What do they want out of this relationship? What life experiences are coloring their interactions? What happened that day, that week, that month, that year to affect how the doctor and patient might relate to one another during a particular visit? What do they need to convey in the moment to be clear about their needs, hopes, and concerns?

There's nothing wrong with a doctor showing a patient their human side; after all, they aren't automatons performing medical tasks and procedures. And there's no reason a patient can't inquire as to how their doctor is doing when they arrive for their visit or if they notice that something seems off. Communicating in this manner is simply us expressing our humanity. I'm not talking about profoundly deep talks where the entirety of one's life is laid on the table, but simply taking an interest in another's well-being beyond health-related checklists, prescriptions, and diagnoses.

Without open and honest communication, no relationship can sustain itself. We'll explore healthy communication as well as common communication pitfalls in chapter 3.

Respect

Respect is easier to understand if we look to its opposite—*disrespect*—because we all pretty much know when someone is being disrespectful. The dictionary says *respect* is to hold someone in high regard, but this is a little misleading. Respect, at its most basic, is treating others with common courtesy and good social manners. It's respecting each other's humanity. That's why the old adage "Respect should be earned, not given" is somewhat inaccurate and can cause an adversarial relationship where none was necessary. We are *all* entitled to respect. This is true for the closest relationships as well as in the everyday interactions we have with others. The simple act of being polite widens the channel for more meaningful interactions.

When it comes to a strong patient-doctor bond, mutual respect is a key component. In addition to respecting each other as human beings, this type of respect manifests in two key areas:

1. Respect for each other's experiences and knowledge

2. Respect for each other's time

Patients are encouraged to ask questions of their doctors to better understand matters concerning their health, but when they question every diagnosis and suggestion the doctor makes because they've researched their symptoms on the internet, they are failing to place value on their doctor's expertise. This lack of respect chips away at this cornerstone quality. Likewise, if a doctor isn't willing to at least briefly consider a patient's brief rundown of research, they aren't respecting the patient's efforts to get to the root of their health issue.

Without this cornerstone firmly in place, there is no avenue for trust, communication, or empathy. How can a patient trust a doctor if that patient doesn't have respect for the doctor's profession and education? How can a doctor expect to effectively communicate with a patient if that doctor doesn't respect the fact that their patient's time is also valuable, and they deserve the doctor's full attention? We will consider these questions and more in chapter 4.

Empathy

Each of the other three cornerstone qualities culminates in empathy, but what exactly is empathy and how do both patients and doctors practice it?

Many physicians strive for a state of "concerned detachment" —the opposite of empathy. In fact, they've often been encouraged to erect emotional barriers to make accurate medical assessments and decisions. Yet patients want and need their doctors to be more empathetic. This leads to a healthcare conundrum.

The argument for detachment is that doctors cannot become personally invested in their patients' troubles and still maintain the objectivity required for proper treatment. But that's looking at empathy in a very narrow way. A leading group from the Society for General Internal Medicine defines *empathy* as "the act of correctly acknowledging the emotional state of another without experiencing that state oneself."[5] So, in other words, empathy isn't necessarily *feeling* what someone else is feeling, but *sensing* another person's emotions and being able to place yourself, at least momentarily, in their frame of reference, thereby gaining the ability to better understand what's going on for them and sympathize with their challenges and struggles.

Keep in mind that for a strong patient-doctor bond, empathy is also a reciprocal action. A patient can also be empathetic to their doctor's feelings, experiences, and challenges. They can

13

understand and acknowledge in the simplest ways that the doctor's daily experiences weigh on them, too.

With trust, respect, and communication, patients and doctors can show that they care about each other as human beings beyond the patient-doctor relationship. In healthcare, empathy is a large and important topic, so I have more to say about it in "Daring to Care" below. Then, in chapter 5, we will continue to explore this quality with the focus on avoiding pitfalls and cultivating empathy in your patient-doctor relationship.

DARING TO CARE

To care for someone is to look after and provide for them; it is recognizing that someone is important to us and so we feel concern for them and take an interest in their well-being. Care is crucial to a solid patient-doctor bond. In fact, it's right there in the name: health*care*. This isn't just about medicine; healthcare is about caring for people, too.

You may have a doctor who doesn't feel like going the extra mile to demonstrate empathy—or doesn't "dare to care," as I like to say. That's unfortunate, but the truth is, it is a little daring to care these days. I empathize: When a doctor sees thirty patients a day, emotionally investing in each one can feel incredibly exhausting. Moreover, showing their human side can make a doctor feel vulnerable when they are supposed to be a stable influence in a patient's life. Likewise, it may be difficult for you to care about your doctor if you simply think of them as a service provider rather than as a person who is doing the best they can do on any given day.

The barriers between patients and doctors need to be chiseled away from both sides because caring isn't one sided. When a doctor knows you care about them as a person and about yourself as a patient and vice versa, you can start moving toward "patient nirvana." Both doctors and patients must show each other that, at the end of the day, we're not all that different. We *need* to care for one another to get the most out of every interaction and appointment. That's what the strengthening of the patient-doctor bond is all about—putting *care* back in healthcare.

It takes time, effort, and dedication to forge a healthy patient-doctor bond. The initial foundation of trust and respect between doctor and patient either deepens or weakens over time. Communication can flow more easily or become encumbered and stilted. And empathy needs to be actively cultivated at each and every encounter, since we can so easily get caught up in ourselves and forget to consider another's experiences and point of view. Moreover, each one of these cornerstones needs the others to create a solid foundation and maintain a solid bond. There is no trust without communication, no communication without respect, and no respect without empathy. No relationship can stand for very long if one of the cornerstones is missing. Likewise, if one of the cornerstones is weak, the whole foundation will eventually collapse.

In the upcoming chapters, we'll explore each of these four cornerstone qualities in depth. We'll discuss the necessary tools to construct each one—and the thoughtless behaviors that can knock them out of place. I want you to come away from the next four chapters with a better understanding of how you and your doctor can meet each other halfway and either establish a bond or strengthen the one you already have.

CHAPTER 2

Trust: Laying the First Cornerstone

"The best way to find out if you can trust somebody is to trust them."

—Ernest Hemingway

Like any good relationship, the foundation of a strong patient-doctor bond is trust. The trust a patient places in their doctor is the assurance and reliance on the doctor's character, ability, integrity, and truth. Without their patients' trust, doctors can't do their jobs properly, patients can't get the quality care they deserve, and there's no hope of building a solid, lasting bond.

Let's say a patient goes to a new doctor. They don't know each other. This is a complete stranger to whom the patient is expected to open up, baring their body, heart, mind, and soul. They wonder, *Can I trust this person with my vulnerabilities? With my health? Can I speak openly without fear of judgment? Will I truly be taken care of?* And what about the doctor? They wonder, *Can I trust this patient to be up-front with me about what's going on for them, not only physically, but mentally and emotionally as well? Can I trust them to take my advice seriously? Can I trust them to be a willing participant in their health and wellness?*

Truly, placing your trust in a person you don't yet have a relationship with takes courage; you're taking a big chance at that very first doctor's appointment with your most valuable asset: your health and wellness. This reminds me of Brené Brown's thought-provoking definition of "trust." To define this cornerstone of the patient-doctor bond, she uses the acronym BRAVING: Boundaries, Reliability, Accountability, Vault (or confidentiality), Integrity, Nonjudgment, and Generosity.[6] That sounds like a tall order, but these qualities comprise a basic code of conduct that's important in any healthy relationship. Hopefully at your first appointment with your new doctor and throughout your relationship with that doctor, you will feel confident that all of these qualities are present. Let's delve deeper into this essential value in your patient-doctor relationship and discuss how to recognize if it is missing or present, as well as how to build it, as Brené Brown says, "in very small moments."

First and Foremost, Trust Your Gut

One of the best ways to determine if someone is trustworthy is by tuning in to how they make you feel on an instinctual level. That's right—checking in with your gut. Have you ever met someone who claimed to have your best interests at heart, but you still had a nagging doubt? That was your gut communicating with your brain that there was more to take into consideration than just the facts as they were presented. As Christopher

Bergland, author of *The Athlete's Way*, explains so clearly, "Visceral feelings and gut instincts are literally emotional intuitions transferred up to your brain via the vagus nerve." The vagus nerve is known as the wandering nerve because it connects the brain to the gut and to many vital organs in between, including the heart. The vagus nerve uses neurotransmitters to prepare the body for both relaxation and fight-or-flight responses to stimuli, and since up to 90 percent of vagus nerve activity is dedicated to sending "gut feeling" signals to the brain, you can trust that a gut feeling—that intuition—you're experiencing is real and is meant to keep you safe.[7]

So be sure to check in with yourself: When you are with your doctor, what is your gut feeling? What is your intuition telling you? How do you feel about this person on an intuitive level? Our gut feelings about people are often spot-on. Our brains rely both on logic and emotions to make decisions, so when deciding if a doctor is worthy of your trust, listen with your whole being. Notice how this person makes you feel and look for subtle clues: Is this person kind to you, really listens when you speak, tries to connect with you on a human level, and appears invested in you, in your health, and in the time you spend in their office?

I'm not suggesting that you withhold important information about your health concerns and challenges while at a doctor's office if you have a feeling this doctor isn't the right one for you—especially if you're there for something serious—but you'll know if this is the doctor with whom you feel you can build a lasting bond. If not, seek a second opinion or continue the search for a primary-care physician you feel you can trust to be there with you for the long haul. There's more on this in chapter 6, so don't stop reading here. There's much more to consider before you run with this advice.

◀ BEHIND THE CURTAIN ▶

I was working as a physician in Los Angeles when a new patient walked through the door. He was an actor who had recently been thrust into the limelight and didn't know how to cope. He had suddenly gone from being a struggling, aspiring actor like so many others in town to being a rising star on a hit television show. His whole world had been turned upside down, and worst of all, he didn't know who he could trust anymore.

I listened attentively to his concerns, empathized with his struggles, and cheered his newfound success. I also told him a little about myself so he could get to know me as a person, and then I offered my best advice for regaining his peace of mind and overall health. As we talked, I could see his face soften and his shoulders relax. Before he left my office that day, he said, "Everyone wants something from me now—my agent, the network, even my fans. But not you. You just want me to be happy and healthy." He understood that my whole focus was on his well-being and that he could trust me to not have my own interests in mind.

A Main Cause of Mistrust in Physicians

A major key barrier to trust is the mistaken idea on the patient's part that there's something in it for the doctor when they prescribe a medication or send the patient for diagnostic tests. Some people believe that there's financial consideration for the doctor when they write a prescription. A patient might even say, "I get it. This is a business." And, yes, it is. That's an inherent problem: Doctors are in a profession that allows them to directly benefit from seeing sick people and helping them get better. Most professions benefit because a person is lacking some sort of skill or time to do something for themselves, and this profession is no different. We virtually all get paid for doing something for others—that's how we make a living.

Still, it's often difficult for a doctor to make a recommendation without a patient thinking there's something in it for them. But let me set the record straight: We *don't* gain financially from the drug companies when we write prescriptions, nor do we get paid to order tests. Only a small number of doctors actually own facilities with imaging equipment. Trust that we're doing testing to arrive at a diagnosis; it's about getting to the root of the problem so that we can help you solve it.

Even though it appears that we derive benefit from illness, we make our living because we take the Hippocratic oath to do no harm. I've given everything I have to make sure that every time I see a patient, I'm changing their life in a positive way. Yes, being a doctor is a job like any other, and we need to make a living like anyone else. But at the end of the day, we don't do it for the money. We do it for the purpose and because health and medicine is what we're passionate about.

Another issue that arises with medications is the patients' perceptions of how the process works. The right medication and right dosage is very patient-specific. Therefore, there usually isn't much value in assuming that a medication that worked for a friend or family member will work for you. But sometimes if a physician prescribes a different medication than the patient was expecting to get, the patient might be concerned that this other medication is being prescribed because it benefits the doctor somehow, when honestly what it usually boils down to is the doctor taking your out-of-pocket expenses into consideration by prescribing based on what your health insurance allows and what medication choices are covered on your formulary. In addition, there are several different medications available within a class that will ensure similar positive out-comes. So I promise that the "good" medicines are not being withheld from you. Your doctor is simply taking all of your needs into account, recognizing that your individual needs may not be met in the same way someone else's might be.

When your doctor spends time typing up your visit and looking at the computer, they are also trying to cross-reference some of the medications you're currently taking to make sure there are no drug interactions. They may also be setting up the medications through your pharmacy, a request that now has to be sent electronically, rather than via a paper script, which also can be a challenge. They're not ignoring you. Rather, they're trying to make the best use of your time so they can make sure you leave with the proper prescription and so they can ask you questions if something in your file doesn't seem congruent with your current plan of treatment.

Can Your Doctor Trust *You*?

Stephen Covey, author of *The Speed of Trust,* says, "We judge ourselves by our intentions and others by their behavior. This is why . . . one of the fastest ways to restore trust is to make and keep commitments—even very small commitments—to ourselves and to others."[8] Have you made a commitment to your doctor to be a "good patient": one who keeps appointments, one who is honest about health concerns and habits, one who follows through on recommendations, and so on? Are you judging whether or not your doctor is to be trusted without judging yourself by the same standards you expect of your doctor?

Just as much as a patient must be able to trust their doctor, a doctor must be able to trust their patient. If a patient doesn't trust their doctor enough to be open and vulnerable, there's a limit to what they can do to help. If you find yourself with-holding information from your doctor during an appointment, you are doing yourself a disservice. There's a good chance your doctor knows you're not telling them the whole story, and that will only erode the bond between you. Opening up is extremely important because your doctor can only work with the infor-mation they are given. Don't limit your doctor. Let your doctor go into this relationship on even ground.

When I'm with a patient, I need to trust that they are being honest with me—not just that they're not lying to me, but also that they're telling me the whole story. Otherwise, I could miss an important sign or symptom. I could misdiagnose a problem. When my gut tells me I don't have the whole story (yes, I listen to my gut, too!), it's very difficult for me to figure out how to make this patient feel better. For example, I've had patients who are struggling with addiction. This is often one of the most difficult things for a patient to admit. Some might tell me out-right, but others try to withhold it. Still, I notice the physical signs of addiction like pinpoint pupils or strange behavior. In some cases, they outright lie even if I have objective evidence, like a urine test. "Oh, I stopped last week," or "Someone must have tampered with that," they tell me. This is incredibly frus-trating. A doctor cannot positively impact a patient's life if they refuse to come clean about what's really going on.

Earning your doctor's trust requires that you allow your doctor a good view of what makes you tick. This takes being vulnerable, open, and honest enough with your doctor so they can get to the core of your truth, whatever it may be. In many cases, it may take a doctor months, even years, to really under-stand you as an individual. Building a trusting relationship takes time and effort. But it is worth it. Because once you have trust, you have a relationship that can withstand almost anything.

◀ BEHIND THE CURTAIN ▶

One of my patients was a big-time hedge fund manager and had been quite successful professionally but struggled in her personal life. Usually, she listened to my advice about shedding some of her excess weight so that she could lead a healthier and potentially longer life, but during one particular appointment, she said, "Look, I get it. My weight is a physical impediment . . ." Then she hesitated. I knew she wanted to say more so I reminded her that she could trust me with whatever was on her mind. She took a breath and went on to say that despite all her success, she felt worthless. She feared she would be single forever. This patient and I had a real heart-to-heart talk then. We talked about her self-worth. We talked about how she had so much to offer another person. Then, we talked about her upbringing and what food means to her. It was incredibly brave of her to be able to admit things like: "I need food to make me happy," and "I feel like I don't deserve a good guy—just critical ones who won't accept me for who I am." The trust she placed in me that day was immense, and it allowed me to help her join a group where she could feel supported and get a handle on her relationship with food.

What Do You Have Trouble Being Honest About?

Get out a pad and paper, and list the top three things you want your doctor to know but would probably withhold because you're too afraid, nervous, or embarrassed to mention it. What might you deny if your doctor asks you about it? For example, have you started smoking again? Have you been drinking alcohol more than a few times a week? Have you been eating snack cakes at midnight? Are you feeling depressed? Do you experience overwhelming bouts of anger from time to time? Are you relying too much on pain medication? Have you and your spouse been fighting more often than usual? These are the types of things, among others, that patients might lie about or not be forthcoming about during their appointments.

To start laying this cornerstone quality in your patient-doctor relationship, look at the top-three things you identified before your next doctor's appointment. When you see your doctor, you might want to say, "You know, there are some things I've been withholding that I want to discuss with you, but I'm a little uncomfortable and I don't know how to go about it." Doing this starts an important dialogue. Your doctor will likely ask, "What do you feel like you can't be honest with me about?" This allows your doctor to dig a little bit deeper into what might be causing your health-related concerns. What you think is a physical medical problem might be due to, or aggravated by, stress, anxiety, or just the normal act of living. So sharing things that you wouldn't otherwise be honest about makes a huge difference in your doctor's ability to help you get to a place of healing.

According to an article in *U.S. News*, a recent survey uncovered that the top reasons for lying to your doctor or omitting important health information were embarrassment or fear of being judged.[9] If you think this might be why you find yourself fibbing a bit, just remember that your doctor's primary goal is not to judge; it's to heal. Besides, no matter how strange you may think your situation is, your doctor has probably heard it before. The same article also notes that some patients may withhold information because they feel there isn't enough time in their appointment, or because they keep waiting for the right opportunity or the right question to be asked. If the doctor doesn't ask, bring up a concern yourself. Steer the conversation that way so the doctor can address your concerns during your appointment. And, to make the most of your time with your doctor so that you don't feel it's necessary to withhold something relevant, see "Making the Most of Your 15 Minutes" on page 70 later in the book.

I also find it helpful for patients to talk about their list of three things with the medical assistant or nurse before they see the doctor. "You know, I want to talk to Dr. X about this issue or experience, but I don't know quite how to approach it." The nurse or medical assistant can get that message conveyed to the doctor so that they can broach the subject without the patient having to initiate the discussion. And then, that's one hurdle we've jumped, taking us closer to the two-way street of patient-doctor trust. We're slowly starting to get back to that perfect zone where you feel like all of your concerns are being addressed.

As I alluded to above, sometimes patients don't want to be honest about things that might cause them to be judged, like smoking for example. I have so many patients who will come in after the new year and tell me, "Doc, this is the year! I'm quitting. I'm done with cigarettes. I'm never smoking again." Then I see them in February, and I ask them how they're doing. "Great," they say. But I smell smoke on them. They're not telling the truth. So I can take three approaches. The first: Shame. But that will get me nowhere. If a patient feels judged, forget about it. They're closed off for good.

The second approach is humor. Sometimes I'll pretend to be outraged. I'll go, "I can't believe someone was smoking next to you! How could someone do that to you? We need to find that person. They should apologize for blowing smoke all over you." And the patient will usually laugh and go, "Alright, alright . . ." They know they can't get anything by me, so they get real.

Sometimes I take a third approach. I tell a story. I tell the patient that my dad was a smoker, too. I tell them, "He tried to quit over and over again, but it never stuck. So I know how difficult that can be. I also know how difficult it was for him to have a son who was a doctor and who would browbeat him. One day, I realized that it wasn't fair of me to treat him like that. He was doing the best he could, and he needed me to be supportive, not judgmental." And then I tell the patient that I hope they feel the same way: "I was patient with my dad, and I will be patient with you, too."

No matter what, it's important for my patients to know that when they're in the four walls of my office, they're in a no-judgment zone. And in that zone, I expect honesty. That's why I like to tell them, in a lighthearted, joking way, "You only have to be honest with two people in your life: your priest and your doctor. Because we're both trying to get you to a better place. We're trying to nurture your soul."

◀ BEHIND THE CURTAIN ▶

I had a patient who was struggling with weight management. He was in his midforties, trying to trim down to his size from his college days, back when he played sports. We discussed various weight-loss strategies over the course of multiple sessions together, but upon each return visit, I'd discover that his weight had only gone up. I figured that maybe he wasn't truly committed to this.

So one day I asked him straight, "What's going on here?" And that's when I learned that his wife—who was struggling with her weight as well—was concerned that if he changed his life, he wouldn't want her anymore.

Ah, there we go. This patient of mine really *did* want to

lose weight to improve his health and happiness, but he also didn't want to alienate his wife. Once I knew that, I was able to ask for her to come in so that we could all sit down and talk. Through an open dialogue with my patient and his wife, we were able to dispel the insecurity and envy and tackle both of their weight management issues together as a team. We never would have come to that resolution if my patient hadn't trusted me enough to open up about his home life. And I know that probably wasn't easy for him.

It's probably not all that easy for you to let your guard down around your doctor either. After all, this is a person you likely barely know. But here's the thing: Opening up to your doctor is absolutely critical to your healthcare. Not only does it help in making the right diagnosis, but it also helps in getting to the real root of the problem in order to take the right approach. An issue like weight management could have multiple different underlying causes—maybe it's that you're miserable at work or maybe you're struggling with your children—and each one requires its own unique treatment plan.

Be Prepared for Some Tough Love

If a doctor is like a member of your family, then you're occasionally going to get some tough love. Because if you can't trust your family to be brutally honest, then who can you trust?

As doctors, we don't always get to tell patients what they want to hear. We have to tell the truth. And sometimes the truth is that a habit or vice—whether it's smoking, drugs, alcohol, or overeating—is leading them down a bad path toward a very unfavorable outcome.

There was a patient of mine who was diabetic and kept coming to see me with blood glucose levels at 300-plus. He would have issues with circulation, and I would say, "It's as simple as taking insulin and following your diet." I'd warn him about the possibility of amputation, but he'd go back to his life and think that it couldn't ever happen to him. A few months later, there was a clot in his foot that required a partial amputation.

As a physician, we've seen it all. And so with our knowledge and our experience, we can see the possible outcomes from miles away. You have to trust that your doctor is going to give it to you straight. Doctors must be there for their patients when they're in denial—and shake them out of it with a healthy dose of real talk. There's no trust without honesty, and there's no honesty like tough love.

Patient Education Builds Trust

I can't stress enough how important it is to me as a physician to make sure that my patients learn what they need to know with regard to their health and health challenges, and they always appreciate the information because it puts their health back in their hands. A study published in the April 2000 edition of *The Journal of Family Practice* revealed that patients who received self-care information directly from their doctor were more satisfied with their care than those who received the same information by mail and those who received no such information.[10] This highlights the importance of direct patient education in building doctor-patient trust, although I don't need a study to know that this is the case because I experience it firsthand in my practice on a daily basis.

I often see patients who have diabetes, which means that we have to do a hemoglobin A1C test every three months to monitor how well we're controlling their blood sugar. The discussions that this monitoring leads to can end up being quite granular—we're literally talking about measuring the amount of sugar on red blood cells. During these types of discussions, the patient might say, "Eh, that's okay, I don't need to know all this." I will shorten my explanation, but I still want them to know the essential information. More often than not, my patients do want to know more. Why? Because this is about their well-being. They might be frustrated because they're not seeing progress and can't understand why, or maybe they've been newly diagnosed with diabetes and they're terrified. Either way, they need to know more because they're invested in their health.

An educated patient is like having a trusty sidekick in this caper that we're pulling off. They're helping the doctor fight any kind of battle that comes their way, whether that's a short-term illness or a long-term disease. They're in it together. And that alone goes a long way toward building trust between a patient and a doctor because it evens the playing field. You no longer have the doctor way up there on his high horse with all that knowledge; you have two people on the same team. Maybe a diabetic patient comes in one day and their A1C number hasn't gone down. That's okay. The patient-doctor team just gets back into the huddle to say, "Alright, what can we do differently to better score against our opponent this time?"

I carry a dry erase board back and forth between patient rooms. People must think it's an odd sight to see, but I like to have it on hand at all times in case a patient has a question that needs a lot of explaining. Maybe it's a patient with gall bladder disease, for example, and I want to make sure that they're really understanding what's going on. So I'll go up to the board like a teacher lecturing a class, and I'll start drawing out the gall bladder, showing where it's nestled into the edge of the liver, and something will click in the patient's head. They get it! And that's all I need. I need them to understand enough about their problem to help me solve it.

In short, when a doctor educates a patient, they gain a trusted partner. That means there's double the manpower attacking a health problem, leading to better overall care. More than that, it means that a patient can leave the doctor's office with their head held high because they know they're directly involved in—and in control of—their healthcare. They're now the captain of their body and soul.

IS DR. GOOGLE IN THE HOUSE?

You wake up one morning and notice that something is off. Maybe you think you have the flu or maybe a part of your body suddenly hurts for no discernible reason. It's 7:00 a.m., your doctor isn't at work yet, and this is the twenty-first century. What do you do? If you're like a lot of other people, you hop online to Google your symptoms.

Look. It's easy. It's cheap. It's readily available at all hours of the day and night. I get it. Dr. Google knows so much. Dr. Google has so many answers. Dr. Google offers so many resources. Honestly, Dr. Google really seems a lot smarter than your primary care doctor.

In myriad ways, technology has radically changed the way healthcare is delivered and practiced. And one of those ways is the sheer volume of information (some valid and some not) at every person's fingertips every day. It only takes an internet connection for you to diagnose yourself—without having to make a doctor's appointment. Some doctors embrace this. They see it as one more educational tool at a patient's disposal that keeps them informed and engaged about their health. But others see it as an annoyance or even a threat to their entire profession. Where does your doctor fit in?

When a patient comes into a doctor's office with pages of research pulled off the internet, their doctor might hear this: "I don't trust you to do your job well enough. I think that I, with the help of technology, can do it better." What I hear is this: "I'm afraid. I'm anxious. I don't feel in control." So instead of pouncing on them for Googling their symptoms, I take a moment to listen. I let them tell me about everything they've found through their research. I take a look through their notes and process their theories. And then I tell them this: "Thank you for sharing your research with me. Let me help you interpret it because your personal health isn't a one-size-fits-all matter."

And that's the truth. Dr. Google doesn't know you. Dr. Google doesn't know that your chest pain is related to the fact that you just bought a new house and started a new job, all while being a newlywed. Dr. Google doesn't know that your asthma flared up because your uncle has cats and you visit him every weekend. Dr. Google doesn't know that you have a headache because you're just hung over after going to a birthday party last night. Every person who has ever Googled their symptoms only to discover they might have cancer (but don't) knows that you can't trust everything you read about your health online.

Technology can only get us so far. Good healthcare requires a human touch, too. Therefore, go ahead and ask Dr. Google for basic information, but rely on your doctor (who probably has Dr. Google's files in their head) to help you do the real healing. The human touch is so key because, yes, you could put all the symptoms in the world into a search engine and possibly come to what might be a diagnosis, but nothing replaces the human mind. Nothing can replace the human ability to look into a person's eyes and see the emotions behind them—because what makes us tick aren't words but feelings.

Meeting Your Doctor in the Middle

After training at the Columbia Presbyterian Medical Center in New York, I went out to California, where patients often turn to alternative methods for healing. Throughout my career, I always yearned to learn more about how to make patients better without my prescription pad, and this seemed like the perfect environment to find patients who might be receptive to methods outside of a pill bottle for treating their health.

Still, despite my preference, there have been plenty of times when I've truly felt that Western medicine offers the most efficacious path to better health. In some cases, patients who prefer alternative medicine have balked at my suggestion to medicate with prescription drugs. For example, one of my patients struggled with high blood pressure, but her reluctance to rely on medication to manage it made it difficult for me to convince her that such medication was essential for her health. In the end, we found a middle ground: she agreed to take the medicine—which was supposed to be taken once per day—three times per week, and only at the lowest dose. While I would have preferred she took the full dose every single day, it gave me peace of mind knowing that, for at least three days a week, she had optimal blood pressure, which would still significantly reduce her risk of a heart attack or a stroke. Maybe I didn't win that battle, but I won the war of keeping her healthy.

It is essential that doctors and patients trust each other enough to meet at the halfway point. It's important to recognize that a doctor's desire to offer the most effective treatments and their patients' desire to control their own healthcare comes from the same place: a desire for better health. Doctors often need to look for the middle ground where their need to treat their patients and those patients' desires to have their wishes respected can coexist, and patients need to be open to that idea as well. Doctors must trust that their patients aren't being obstinate for the sake of being obstinate, and patients must trust that the treatments their doctors suggest are offered out of a desire to give them every possible chance to be healthier. Trust can't be an all-or-nothing game. It takes compromise. As doctors, we don't always get what we want. But if we do our jobs right, the patient still gets what they need.

BUILDING TRUST CHEAT SHEET

✓ When you know that your doctor is in good standing with your state's medical board, trust that your doctor is qualified to help you make important healthcare decisions. It's okay to ask for alternative suggestions, if available, but understand that your doctor is using years of accumulated knowledge and wisdom to offer you a treatment plan.

✓ Have faith that your doctor chose this profession because they have an aptitude for medical care and truly do want to help improve people's lives, not just make a "quick buck."

✓ Go ahead and search your symptoms on the internet, but remember that this information can be inaccurate or misleading. If you are experiencing troublesome symptoms, always seek counsel from your doctor, and keep the "But Google said . . ." to a minimum during your visit.

✓ Always tell your doctor the full truth. Withholding information from your doctor can negatively impact your doctor's ability to help you. Being honest with your doctor, even about the most embarrassing things, will build your doctor's trust in you.

From Doctor to Doctor

Here are some approaches that have worked for me in my practice to help deepen the trust between my patients and me. Maybe you will find them helpful as well for building trust and solidifying the patient-doctor bond you have with your patients.

- After greeting a patient, I explicitly tell them that my office is a no-judgment zone and that they can trust me not to judge them when they confide in me. I still practice "tough love" when necessary, but I do so without making them feel bad about themselves for "falling off the wagon" or not practicing healthy habits.

- I make an effort to find common ground to help my patients let their guard down around me. It might be sports. It might be our favorite restaurants in town. It might be silly stories from when we were kids. This lets them know I'm human, too, with similar vulnerabilities and strengths. It's a sort of "Trust me, we're all in this together" approach—and it's the God's honest truth.

- If my gut tells me or my observations show me that a patient is lying to me, I use either humor or a personal anecdote to get them to come clean. I never shame my patients.

- I take time to educate my patients on their health issues to ease their concerns and frustration and build their trust in my recommendations. I want to know that my patient understands exactly what's going on with their bodies so that they feel empowered to do something about it and take the necessary steps to get healthy.

CHAPTER 3

Communication: Exchanging Information for Mutual Benefit

"A pair of kidneys will never come to the physician for diagnosis and treatment. They will be contained within an anxious, fearful, wondering person, asking puzzled questions about an obscure future, weighed down by the responsibilities of a loved family, and with a job to be held, and with bills to be paid."

—Dr. Philip Tumulty

As a physician, I can think of no other place that healthy, open communication is more important than in a doctor's office. The information that's exchanged during a doctor's visit surely falls into the category of "crucial conversations." In the bestselling book *Crucial Conversations*, the authors define this type of conversation as "a discussion between two or more people where (1) the stakes are high, (2) opinions vary, and (3) emotions run strong."[11] Now, when it comes to your health, the stakes are always high, and, yes, your opinion of what's best for you may differ from your doctor's, and it's likely that if something serious is going on, your emotions are strong. But even if all of your interactions with your doctor don't include all three of these factors, what you say to your doctor and what your doctor says to you *is* crucial information.

A 2010 article in *The Ochsner Journal* explains that open communication between patient and doctor not only promotes trust but better health overall. A patient whose doctor is communicative and trustworthy is more likely to feel empowered to choose to follow that doctor's prescribed plan of treatment, and a doctor whose patient is open and truthful about their concerns allows the doctor to find the most viable and effective treatment possible.[12] When a doctor and patient are on the same page, the likelihood of continued health and/or regaining one's health increases. Read on to learn how to lay this integral cornerstone in your patient-doctor relationship so that, in the end, everyone wins.

A Healthcare Problem

A doctor's visit isn't a social call, but it is a social exchange between two people in which information is shared over a common bridge: your health. Once social niceties are exchanged, succinctly communicating the reason for your visit, your health-related concerns, and whatever might be applicable to your current situation (for example, how long you've had an issue, what's going on in your home or work life that might be contributing, etc.) will give your doctor a platform from which they can effectively share health-related information with you and make an accurate diagnosis. This leads to better overall care. When patients properly understand their doctors, they are more likely to acknowledge problems with their health, modify their behavior, and follow medication schedules and treatment plans.[13]

Unfortunately, communication—that is, a lack of communication and miscommunication—is often at the root of many problems in healthcare. Doctors and patients cannot form a real and lasting connection unless they feel as if they're being heard by the other at each appointment. Patients often complain that they don't feel like their doctor understands what they need or get what's going on with them and feel helpless as a result. The culprit is likely miscommunication because the last thing a doctor wants is for their patient to feel helpless, especially when they've come to their office for a well-communicated, problem-solving interaction. We all want to conclude our appointments feeling like we're on the same page. Interestingly, studies have shown that doctors tend to overestimate their communication skills, while surveys of patients have consistently shown a desire for better communication with their doctors. In fact, most complaints about doctors are related to issues with their communication skills, not their competency.[14] Fortunately, this is an area that can be improved with a little extra effort.

In the article "Doctor-Patient Communication: A Review," published in the *Ochsner Journal,* the authors state that "the 3 main goals of current doctor-patient communication are creating a good interpersonal relationship, facilitating exchange of information, and including patients in decision making." As with all interpersonal relationships, barriers to effective doctor-patient communication may crop up. Patients may feel fearful or resistant to a doctor's prescribed method of treatment, or they may have unrealistic expectations about what their doctor can do for them. Doctors, on the other hand, may feel over-worked, fearful of patient backlash if their treatment doesn't have the desired effect, or concerned that their recommendations will not be followed. This might lead to close-mindedness on the doctor's part, wherein the doctor doesn't allow a patient to voice their concerns, and to resistance on the patient's part to sharing their concerns or taking the doctor's advice. This is a lose-lose situation.

Recognizing these potential roadblocks in your relationship with your doctor is the first step toward healthy communication. Simply put, both patient and doctor must be consciously willing not only to share anything they feel may be pertinent to a successful treatment but also to listen to what the other side has to say. If you feel your doctor is withholding information or being unreceptive to your concerns, be willing to speak up for yourself. Once you feel your doctor has become open to what you have to say, be willing to do the same for them.

What Is Healthy Communication?

Why is it such a struggle for people to communicate effectively with one another? Why can't we just sit down and say exactly what's on our mind and be understood and heard by the other person? We're being clear and concise, aren't we? Could it be that we need to improve how we communicate?

Healthy communication is clear, honest, targeted, and accurate. It involves both speaking *and* listening—and being fully present. The speaker has the responsibility of making sure that they are heard and understood, and the listener has the responsibility to ask questions or ask for information to be repeated if they don't understand what the speaker has said. In order to do this, both parties need to be mindful of what they are saying and hearing. This means putting aside all assumptions and unrelated thoughts for the moment. In fact, I feel that practicing mindfulness while you are with your doctor and vice versa is at the core of a productive doctor's visit. Mindfulness means being fully aware in the present moment, and therefore, mindful communication means that you are completely focused on your conversation as both speaker and listener.

When I think about healthy patient-doctor communication, I picture it to be almost like a beautiful ballet in which all the movements are perfect. The patient listens to the doctor as much as the doctor listens to the patient. The result is a masterpiece of communication that both parties can feel good about and leaves everyone involved feeling fulfilled, inspired, and hopeful.

The Guessing Game

Doctors sometimes need to put on their detective hat when speaking with a patient. I've been in situations where patients come in with a health complaint and a list of symptoms, which I could use to arrive at a diagnosis, but when I press for more, I discover that the patient hadn't told me everything—not necessarily because they were being dishonest or intentionally keeping something from me, but because they weren't thoroughly or clearly communicating what I needed to know. Finding out this "hidden" information makes a huge difference in my ability to help. This would not have been possible if I didn't make two-way communication with my patient during the exam a top priority. However, we would have more quickly arrived at a solution if my patient hadn't left out important details in the first place. I admit that a patient may think that something's not important enough to mention, so it's really up to the doctor to ask questions to get a full picture. Doctors aren't going to intuitively know, for instance, that you just started using a new laundry detergent that is the potential cause of your rash if you don't tell them. We aren't mind readers.

In the same way doctors are not mind readers, patients aren't translators. They can't listen to medical jargon and automatically translate it into lay terms so that they can take action based on what their doctor has said. If a patient has to guess what a doctor means when they say, "Your echocardiogram shows that you have some mitral regurgitation that needs to be addressed," something is faulty with how the doctor is communicating. In a case like this, I would explain to the patient not only what an echocardiogram is (essentially an ultrasound of the heart; an inside picture of what's going on), but I would also explain that it showed that the blood flow is backing up (hence the term "regurgitation") in his or her mitral valve—one of the four valves in the heart. I would also clearly explain our next steps. Not all doctors take the time to speak in lay terms like this, and not all patients request clarification. This is another lose-lose situation that can be turned around when both parties make exchanging straightforward information a priority.

◀ BEHIND THE CURTAIN ▶

Many years ago, one of my patients was newly diagnosed with asthma. I prescribed two different inhalers and explained that one was for rapid action for acute attacks and the other for chronic action and inflammation in the airways for daily use. She nodded to everything I said, and I believed she was ready to manage her asthma with the medication and advice I had given her. However, when she came for her follow-up a few weeks later, she wasn't progressing the way I had expected her to. We should have seen *some* improvement after a few weeks on the medication.

When I asked if she had been using her daily inhaler regularly, she squirmed a bit and said, "Truthfully, Dr. Redcross, I've only been using it if I feel like I need it because I wasn't sure which was which."

"Why didn't you call to check?" I asked.

"Oh," she replied, "I didn't want to bother you. I figured it could wait until now."

Rather than become upset or frustrated that she hadn't followed my instructions, I gave her a smile and said, "You can never bother me, especially when it comes to your health."

At that point, I realized that although I had communicated the inhalers' purposes at our previous appointment, she hadn't really understood exactly when to use them, how often to use them, and why she was using them (in other words, why I had prescribed them). I didn't explain to her at that initial appointment that the inhalers would be two different colors, to help emphasize which was for everyday use and which was for acute flare-ups.

I went over with her in detail how, when, and why to use the inhalers, and when she nodded in response, I said, "Okay, great, you understand, but now it's your turn to explain it to me!" When she repeated back the information I had given her, I was 100 percent certain that this patient would be able to use the medication to get her asthma under control.

Listening Is Communicating

Good communicators are good listeners. When it comes to listening, I like to think of the words "earth" and "heart." When we are grounded in the earth (all that is) and approach the world from our heart, we are reminded of the important gift found in those two words: "ear." It's a reminder to me to listen. I believe that one of the best ways doctors show they are good communicators is actually by *not* talking. You've probably heard the old adage "We only have one mouth and two ears." It pretty much means that we're supposed to listen twice as much as we talk. Many times I'm able to get to a diagnosis—or at least arrive at a good understanding of what's going on for that patient—by just plainly listening. I don't only listen to what my patient is saying, but how they're saying it. Are their facial expressions changing? Are they becoming more anxious? More relaxed? Happier? Smiling? Frowning?

Incredibly, research has found that physicians interrupt patients after approximately twenty-three seconds into a visit.[15] They simply don't allow the patient to complete presenting their complaints before jumping in, which can result in their missing important information that the patient may not bring up later. I get it, with just fifteen minutes devoted to each visit and so many things interfering with the schedule, a doctor wants to get straight to the point. That's understandable, but a doctor who wants to show that they care must remain engaged with the patient who's sitting in front of them and deserving of their time. When a doctor actively participates in the conversation by listening, they convey a sense of approachability, making their patients comfortable enough to open up.

If your doctor is an interrupter, ask your doctor for a few minutes so you can explain what's been going on for you. A doctor who wants to have a solid patient-doctor relationship will give you the time to get into your issue without jumping to a diagnosis.

Of course the onus is mostly on doctors to be active listeners, but patients also need to practice the art of listening when their doctor is speaking to them. It's understandable that a patient may have many questions and concerns going on in their mind, and they're not quite present when the doctor is speaking. It's important to make an effort to listen to your doctor with your full attention to get the most from your appointment. Studies show that up to 80 percent of medical information that patients receive is immediately forgotten and nearly half of the retained information is actually incorrect.[16] That's pretty alarming. Don't be one of those patients. Your listening skills are essential for accurately remembering what your doctor says. If you feel you can't retain it all, take notes. If you know that you and your doctor will be discussing a lot of important health-related information at a particular visit, consider bringing along a companion (four ears are even better at listening than two!).

Clear Explanations Are Key

A patient comes in to receive a diagnosis that needs to be discussed. Their doctor says that they have anemia but that everything will be fine. Assuming that their patient knows what anemia is, they fail to properly explain the diagnosis, leaving the patient confused and concerned. Here's another example: A patient has been having pain in the upper right portion of her abdomen and has a sonogram that reveals small polyps in the gallbladder, not gallstones. The doctor says the polyps are probably nothing to be concerned about, again, assuming that the patient knows what a polyp is. *Anemia* and *polyps* are words that sound simple and seem common enough, but when it comes to a diagnosis, a doctor cannot assume that their patient really understands what they mean. And because the words do sound simple, the patient may feel foolish asking for further explanation.

When you are visiting with your doctor, make sure you understand what your doctor is telling you. It's perfectly okay for you to ask questions for clarification. Ask your doctor to slow down and keep their language as simple as possible. Sometimes, your doctor just needs to be reminded that this information is completely new to you. I encourage you to repeat back to your doctor what they have told you in your own words so that your doctor can be certain you've heard them and fully understand them.

In my practice, my goal is to have every patient leave armed with more knowledge than when they came in. They should not only understand what happened during our visit but they should also have a firm enough grasp on their diagnosis or treatment plan that they can explain it to someone else. As I mentioned earlier, I use a dry erase board to illustrate what's going on with an organ or other body part so that my patients get a really clear picture (pun intended) of their diagnosis and what's happening in their body as a result of their condition. I'm no Picasso so my patients and I often have a good laugh, but I also know that this exercise is really driving home for them what I'm trying to explain.

I also make sure my patients can answer three important questions before they leave my office. The Ask Me 3® educational program, which is run by the Institute for Healthcare Improvement, outlines three questions that every patient should be able to answer at the end of their visit.[17] They are:

1. What is my main problem?

2. What do I need to do?

3. Why is it important for me to do this?

When you can accurately answer these three questions when you leave your doctor's office, you know that you and your doctor have aced the communication category.

Of course I've placed a lot of emphasis here on the importance of a doctor providing their patients with clear explanations, but patients have some explaining to do as well. What brings you to the doctor's office that day? It's called a chief complaint. By the way, this may be different from the main problem you take away from your visit. Your chief complaint might be coughing, but your main problem as diagnosed by your doctor is bronchitis.

If you're able to convey your chief complaint to your doctor's office even before the visit, your doctor will be one step ahead of the game when they enter the exam room. When it comes to explaining what's going on with you, I have two more pieces of advice to share in the next section.

◀ BEHIND THE CURTAIN ▶

Years ago, I was working in a large practice with several really great doctors, and often, if the doctor a patient wanted to see was unavailable, they would be given the option to see another doctor in the practice. This happened in the case of a patient I had seen on a few occasions before I found out that I wasn't the doctor she had initially hoped to see.

On this particular occasion, I needed to speak with her about blood in her urine, which had showed up in her urine test. I asked a few questions, which she answered, but when I started to ask more female-specific questions, she cut me short. "Oh, let's just go over the basics because I don't really feel comfortable talking with you about this topic."

I was a bit taken aback and said, "I understand how this can be uncomfortable for you and we can certainly make an appointment for you to see one of the female doctors, but tell me, why have you been scheduling appointments with me all this time?"

"Well, originally, I had wanted to see Dr. Karen, but then I got you, and it's really been fine because you're not how I imagined a male doctor would be, but I still prefer to talk about woman things with a woman. I didn't want to hurt your feelings."

"I'm so glad you are telling me this now," I assured her. "For us to continue having a patient-doctor relationship, it's really important that you feel comfortable enough with me to tell me anything concerning your health and well-being. For a *guy* doctor," I said with a smile to add some levity, "I promise I'm a pretty good listener and problem-solver. But of course, I can make a referral or send in one of the nurses to get you in to see one of the female doctors as soon as possible."

The patient seemed to be weighing her options in her mind, and I reminded her that whatever decision she made it was okay with me. I assured her that whatever worked best for her to keep her happy and healthy was what I wanted, but also stressed in a pleasant manner that open communication on both of our parts would be necessary for us to continue the doctor-patient relationship we had formed over the course of her previous visits. Ultimately, she chose a female doctor, which I think was the best for her. If she wasn't comfortable communicating with me, I would not be able to properly support her ongoing needs for optimal health.

Too Much and Too Little . . .

Imagine that a patient visits their doctor with a laundry list of issues: Their right earlobe twinges, the big toe on their right foot cramps while jogging, they've been getting a rash on their right elbow since they were little, their stomach hurts, and they can't deal with the stress at work. When a patient shows up with a binder full of problems, it's not uncommon for a doctor to think something like, *Oh boy. I've got a waiting room full of patients, and I have a copy of* War and Peace *to get through!* Of course your doctor cares about your concerns, but only so much can be accomplished in one visit—or at least this list needs to be prioritized.

In this laundry list of complaints, what stands out to you as the most important? Without actually seeing the rash, it would seem that the top priority would be that stomachache. That doesn't mean you shouldn't mention the rash, your elbow, and the stress, of course, but it's up to your doctor to address your chief complaint and decide if those other complaints are relevant or not. When my patients bring in a list, I take the list and run down it myself, knocking things out as much as possible as I go so we can hone in on the most serious issues that need to be addressed at that appointment. I speak aloud each item on the list and offer some of my preliminary advice as necessary and then physically check items off, which helps the patient know that they've been heard.

As I mentioned, your doctor simply can't solve everything at once. In a fifteen-minute time slot, only so much can be accomplished. (Later in chapter 4, you'll get an up-close look at what should ideally happen during these "magical" fifteen minutes.) I would *never* tell a patient to ignore a health issue or to not voice a concern. Remember, we want you to trust us enough to be completely open and honest. But you should understand that if you have many unrelated health complaints that don't fall into the emergency category, your doctor will need to treat your most pressing concerns at this visit and you'll need to schedule another visit to address other things.

Make your list, and then circle the most acute, urgent things that absolutely need to be addressed in this visit (see "The Top-4 Complaints to Mention First and Never Leave Off Your List" below). Let's deal with those first. Then, if your appointment is winding down, briefly mention your other concerns again, and if your doctor determines that they aren't connected to your main complaint, schedule a separate appointment.

THE TOP-4 COMPLAINTS TO MENTION FIRST AND NEVER LEAVE OFF YOUR LIST

Always tell your doctor if you are experiencing any of the following health concerns regardless of why you scheduled your appointment *before* you mention any other health issues you are having:

1. Mental health complaints, such as depression and anxiety

2. Cardiac complaints, such as chest pain, chest heaviness, and chest tightness

3. Pulmonary complaints, such as breathing difficulties, shortness of breath, and loss of breath

4. Abdominal complaints, such as constipation, diarrhea, cramping, blood in the stool, and changes in the stool

While too much information can impede effective communication, so can too little information. To get the most out of your doctor's visit, you need to be very specific with what's going on. Does the following scenario sound at all familiar to you?

ME: "What brings you in today?"

PATIENT: "I don't really know, but I feel like I need to be seen."

ME: "Okay, what's wrong?"

PATIENT: "I'm in pain."

ME: "Where do you feel pain?"

PATIENT: "All over."

ME: "And how long have you felt this pain?"

PATIENT: "I don't know."

There's not a lot I can do with that information. As a patient, it's important to keep track of your symptoms so that you can articulate exactly what's going on with your health. The more details you provide your doctor, the better—and quicker—they can help. As an example, with diabetic patients, I often ask that they keep a blood sugar diary to document what and when they're eating. This additional information comes in handy during their regular hemoglobin A1C tests. And this goes for all patients: Documenting pertinent information will allow your doctor to more effectively and efficiently help manage your health. Whether you call it a diary or journal, you'd be surprised at how effective it is.

THE BENEFITS OF KEEPING A JOURNAL

A journal is a method of communicating with your future self and your doctor. We can't possibly remember everything we eat, drink, and experience in a day (hey, we have to make room in our heads for the fun stuff, too!), so keeping a record is a way for you and your doctor to connect the dots and potentially make a connection between different symptoms or get control of the symptoms you experience. I stress the need for this with my insulin-dependent diabetic patients. For example, if I see that your blood sugars are really high in the morning, then I know that your insulin dose at midday or at bedtime needs to be adjusted.

A food diary is great for weight management, too. I know it's not easy to keep detailed records, but there are lots of smartphone apps out there that help to track your diet and also track the calories along the way. Another thing I like for my patients to journal is their mood. How did they do that day? What sort of things were going on? Our mood has an effect on our health and vice versa, so this is important information to share with your doctor, too, especially if you are in the midst of challenges.

When a patient keeps these types of records and shares it with me at our appointment, pointing out anything out of the ordinary, they are arming me with a lot of really useful information to help them get to a place of feeling good.

Feedback Welcome

Asking for feedback is something doctors don't do enough of. There would be nothing strange about it if your doctor, at the end of your visit, simply asked, "Was I able to meet your expectations today?" or "Do you feel confident that you understand our plan?" Has your doctor ever asked you these types of questions? Even if you only have positive feedback for your doctor, questions regarding your satisfaction can help you feel like your doctor cares about you as a human being and not as an appointment.

Even if your doctor doesn't ask for it, I encourage you to offer feedback at the end of your visit and urge you to speak up if you feel that your doctor hasn't met your expectations at that particular visit. Would you like more time with your doctor because you're not accomplishing enough in fifteen minutes— or even less? Tell them that. They might be able to schedule two slots for you. Unless you tell your doctor the things that will make you happier as a patient, they'll never know, and there will never be improvement.

This is especially important if you have a concern about your doctor's staff. Your physician is mostly in the back of the office, busy with patients, and unaware of what's going on up front. We don't know if you weren't greeted or if you were treated rudely by the receptionist. And all of this affects how patients perceive their visit, and therefore how they rate their doctor.

I know that patients are sometimes nervous to report issues to their doctor because they're not sure how they'll take it. If a nurse has been with a doctor for thirty years, they don't want to say, "Hey, you should have gotten rid of her twenty-nine years ago. She's horrible." (Also, maybe don't phrase it like that.) Maybe they're worried that they'll be insulting. Maybe they think that their feedback will fall on deaf ears. All the more reason why a doctor should solicit that feedback. Anything that you think is affecting your ability to see your doctor and get the care you deserve needs to be conveyed to them. Don't be afraid to honestly communicate your feedback.

STRENGTHENING COMMUNICATION CHEAT SHEET

✓ When you make your doctor's appointment, be clear with the staff about your reason for making the appointment so that your doctor knows what your chief complaint is. This gives your doctor a chance to put on their "thinking cap" even before the enter the examination room.

✓ Before your appointment, make a list of what you want to talk to your doctor about. This list can include physical, mental, and emotional issues, all of which may be affecting your health. Also, make a list of specific questions you would like answered. Make two drafts—one where you write down everything you can think of, which you will keep, and the other for your doctor that prioritizes your concerns in order of severity or importance. If you type this list up, you can actually hand your doctor the paper.

✓ Track information related to your health issues in a journal or diary.

✓ Mindfully listen to your doctor with the expectation that you will clearly understand what they are saying. If you don't understand or you need additional information, always ask questions—no matter how silly or ignorant you think they might sound.

✓ Repeat back to your doctor what you think they said so they can confirm that you're on the same page.

✓ Take notes during your visit so that you can remember what was communicated.

▨▨▨▨▨▨From Doctor to Doctor ▨▨▨▨

Here are some approaches that have worked for me in my practice to help enhance communication between my patients and me. Maybe you will find them helpful as well for strengthening the level of communication and solidifying the patient-doctor bond you have with your patients.

- One of the biggest things impeding a doctor's ability to listen today is the use of an electronic medical record. It can be a real distraction when we should be focusing on our patients. Sure we need to document during the appointment, but I always pick up my head, look at my patient, and use eye contact to show that I'm actually in this conversation with them. In the same way I notice my patient's nonverbal cues, I also use nonverbal clues like nodding my head and using facial expressions to let them know that I'm listening to them—not just hearing the words they speak, but really listening with my whole being. That doesn't mean I don't take a moment to take notes or review their records (I have to in order to be able to keep up with the paperwork), but I do try to find a good balance between looking at my patient and looking at my screen.

- I avoid medical jargon, but that doesn't mean I don't use correct medical terms. I explain everything in terms that anyone can understand and define all medical terms for my patients. I also purposely slow down when I speak, not in a condescending way but in a way I can be sure I'm clearly communicating what I need to say. I keep my language simple and human. I always ask my patients if they understand what I'm saying. I don't assume anything or leave any room for miscommunication.

- I use the Ask Me 3® technique to check if my patient has fully understood our encounter (see page 46).

- I always follow up with my patients. One of the biggest questions patients have is "How will I know my test results?" A patient should never have to wonder that. Some doctors have a policy that if you don't hear anything, assume that everything's fine. But that doesn't sit well with most people, and why would it? That's not effective communication, and it's not giving the patients peace of mind.

- When I greet my patient in the examination room, I ask, "How was your visit up-front today? I assume everything was fine." Chances are good that everything was fine. But if you start to see eye rolls, that's when you know. It all comes out: "I never have a good experience," they'll say. Or maybe, "Oh, you know, they're busy." And, yes, a doctor's staff is busy, but it should never be to the point that a patient feels ignored or mistreated. I try to get details from the patient so it's not just some vague complaint that I'll have difficulty addressing. Afterward, it's important to speak to the office staff to find out what went wrong with that particular patient and if any patients might have a similar complaint. This can be a really touchy subject for us doctors (especially ones like me who want everyone to be happy), but we need to listen to our patients' complaints and let our staff explain their side of the story.

- Because some patients don't feel comfortable complaining or making suggestions for improvement, I like to keep a suggestion box for my patients to leave comments anonymously and honestly. This helps me understand exactly what my patients are feeling, how they're perceiving the service at my office, and how their experience can be improved.

CHAPTER 4

Respect: Treating Each Other with Honor and Dignity

"One of the most sincere forms of respect is actually listening to what another has to say."

—BRYANT H. MCGILL

Respect is a core piece of any relationship. In the most literal sense, *respect* is a feeling of deep admiration for someone, whether you're moved by their achievements or their attributes. In a patient-doctor bond, that's exactly what we need to do: we need to admire each other. It doesn't have to be a deep admiration—especially not right away—but we must be able to communicate through our words and our actions: "I choose you. I honor you."

There are many ways to show respect for another person. You can acknowledge their station in life, their talents, knowledge, opinions, and experiences. You can be mindful of their time—not leaving them waiting and not valuing your needs and wishes over theirs. And on a more basic level, you can treat them as no more and no less than who they are—a fellow human being. In his book, *The Top Ten Laws of Respect*, N. Taiwo points out three different types of respect and labels them *human respect, positional respect,* and *earned respect.*[18] Within these categories are many subjective nuances based on personal and societal values. Clearly, respect is a multifaceted concept that each of us needs to define for ourselves while keeping in mind what respect means to the people we are interacting with and what it means to our society as a whole.

In this chapter, we'll dive into the third cornerstone of the patient-doctor bond and explore the manifestations of respect in the patient-doctor relationship with perspectives on how patients and doctors can better show admiration for one another. We'll also talk about all the ways we get under each other's skin—from doctors failing to pay attention to their patients to patients brushing off their doctor's recommendations to the most frustrating thing of all: that long wait in the waiting room.

How Respect Manifests in the Patient-Doctor Relationship

As studies show, respect manifests itself in many ways in the patient-doctor relationship. In the *Journal of Medical Ethics,* in the 2009 article, "Understanding Respect: Learning from Patients," the following elements were identified regarding respect: attention to needs, empathy, care, autonomy, recognition of individuality, information provision, and dignity.[19] Doctors must be attentive to a patient's needs—not ignore their requests or invalidate their concerns. Patients must consider their doctor's advisement, yet still feel like they're in control of their healthcare decisions. Doctors must show dignity for their patients by not talking down to them or assuming that they don't know what they're talking about. Patients must feel that they have their doctor's full attention and are their primary priority—at least for a period of time.

That reads like a tall order, but in reality, this is what a doctor needs to do at every visit. When patients feel that they're being made aware of all the options available to them and that these options are being offered with their own unique needs in mind, they will feel empowered by their doctor's show of respect. In turn, they will offer their doctor the same show of respect in other ways, which builds or reinforces this essential cornerstone in the relationship.

◀ BEHIND THE CURTAIN ▶

At my concierge medical practice, I encourage my patients to reach out to me with a text or phone call if they have a concern they don't think can wait until our next appointment. After working in all different types of healthcare settings, I chose this approach for my private practice because this is the style that works best for my patients and me.

Some of my patients often fly into town for acting or signing gigs. They might come in for a checkup, or if they're not feeling well while they are preparing for their performance, they reach out to me. Keep in mind, this might be late at night, but they know that no matter the hour, I'll be there to care for them.

One morning, I heard from one of these patients, who said, "Hey, I could have used you last night. But it was one a.m., and I didn't want to bother you. I know you have small kids. And I figured it could wait until morning." Honestly, I was floored. This particular patient happened to be a pretty well-known celebrity who always has his needs met, who is basically told whatever he wants to hear all day every day. Yet he was thinking about what was best for *me*. He was being respectful of my time and what I have going on in my life. I felt honored to be on the receiving end of his respect. Still, I reminded him that his being able to call me at 1 a.m. was precisely the reason I was his doctor!

Keep in mind that I recognize it isn't feasible for doctors in a large general practice to give out their personal numbers to their patients. Some might to a few select patients with whom they have a long-standing bond, but it's generally not the rule. My decision to establish a concierge practice included this type of one-on-one service, and some doctors might cringe at the idea of patients being able to call them any time of night. Fortunately, I know that my patients respect me enough to only call me personally when a real need arises.

Respect for a Doctor's Profession

On a few occasions I've had a patient walk into my office, and I've felt it right away: This guy (or gal) has already made up his (or her) mind about me, and he (or she) doesn't care what I have to say. On the surface, it's a lack of respect for my profession as a doctor, but oftentimes, there's something else going on, whether that's a feeling of entitlement or a know-it-all attitude. Or (and this is more common that you might think) the patient has been burned so many times and has become so jaded that they've lost all respect for the medical community. Those are difficult waters to navigate. How can I do my job well if my patient is turned off before we've even gotten started? Depending on the situation, I take a certain approach to earning back that patient's respect.

With a jaded patient, I admit that, as human beings, doctors make mistakes. We're afforded a few mulligans, but after a certain point, some patients might get turned off. There were just too many times when a doctor said they'd call with the lab results and didn't or gave the wrong diagnosis. And so now that patient has written off all doctors everywhere. I get it. They've been given no reason to respect or trust doctors—and certainly no reason to trust or respect me, a doctor they've just met. So I tell it to them straight: I say, "Look, I know that something has happened in your healthcare past to make you distrustful of my profession. But you don't know me yet. How can you be upset with me already? I'm not asking you to trust me and like me right away. But I'm asking you to give me a shot." I know that these patients have heard it all before, so I don't flood them on the first day. I just ask for them to give me the benefit of the doubt. And then we try to get to a better place someday, one that includes mutual respect.

There's also the entitled patient. For example, a wealthy or powerful patient may come off as disrespectful, believing that their time is more important, their life is more important, and their needs and desires are more important than mine and others in the waiting room. The only way I can get a person like that to respect my role as their doctor, advisor, and confidant is by not letting my frustration show, being patient with them, and proving myself through my work and care.

The know-it-all patient also takes some work. Perhaps a patient has a doctor in their family and thinks that they know everything about diseases and medicine that there is to know. No matter what I say, they always know more than I do. It doesn't matter that I went to medical school and have been doing this for years. Instead of dismissing them, I say, "Let me tell you my thoughts first, and then you can go talk to the doctor in your family or tell me what you think." I have to respect their view of their care and their own knowledge, but they have to respect that they came to me for a reason.

And if none of that works? Then sometimes we have to accept that maybe this just isn't a match. If you don't respect me as a doctor, then there's a limit to how much I can help you.

If you recognize yourself in one of these descriptions, it's important to acknowledge to yourself that maybe you aren't giving your doctor a fighting chance. Start by respecting the simple fact that your doctor wants to help you and then allow that to grow into full-fledged respect as your doctor earns it by showing you they respect you as a patient.

Respect for a Patient's Profession or Pursuits

Of course, respect goes both ways; it can't be one-sided. Just as my patient needs to respect my profession, I need to respect theirs, too. As a doctor, I'm no better than any patient who comes into my office. That's why I always ask my patients what they do or did for a living. Knowing a person's professional journey is a pathway to admiration. I also keep in mind that some patients may be stay-at-home moms or dads or are still in school. I try not to make assumptions, and if that's the case, I know they are still making a contribution to the world in whatever way they've chosen. In other words, I respect their choices and admire their passions and pursuits.

Sometimes when I ask a patient what they do for work, they'll wave me away, thinking that what they do isn't all that important. A patient might say, "You know, I do such and such, and it might not make a ton of money or be a big deal, but I like it." And I say, "Are you kidding me? Liking what you do is a very big deal!" If a patient doesn't feel inspired by their job or their role in life, as if they owe themselves more, I feel for them. I respect that they are at this place in life where they're just not content, and in cases like that I offer encouragement. Likewise, when someone is pursuing their dreams, I commend and honor that.

Give your doctor a chance to know what makes you tick professionally and personally. Allow them to see you as more than just a patient. It's an important reminder for us.

It's About Time: Respecting Schedules

Let's say you're a financial specialist and you've scheduled a meeting to discuss a new investment account with a couple who will be coming upon retirement in ten years. The meeting to discuss this investment has been scheduled for over a week, but when the time comes to have the meeting, the couple doesn't show up. Five minutes go by, and you still haven't heard from them. After another five minutes go by, you're beginning to feel frustrated. By the half-hour mark, you're downright livid. You call the couple to find out where they are only to discover they had gotten caught up in something and had forgotten the meeting. While their message to you may have been unintentional, it's crystal clear that the couple just wasn't respecting you or your time.

One of the major ways we show respect to others is by honoring their time. If a patient is late for their doctor's appointment, the doctor feels frustrated and disrespected—just as the patient feels when the doctor is running behind schedule.

Let's talk about time from your point of view first. When you make an appointment to see your doctor, it's usually because you have a complaint or a problem. You're concerned and you have to go through the process of finding a doctor (if you don't already have one), calling the office, and securing the next available appointment. Once you do get a slot on your doctor's electronic medical record, it's just for fifteen minutes, and it's likely preceded by a good amount of idle time in the waiting room. So when you finally do get to see your doctor, you deserve your doctor's full attention, and your doctor needs to be respectful of the fact that you made a lot of effort making an appointment and spent a lot of time waiting to be seen. There's not a lot that your doctor can do to make your wait time any shorter, but a good doctor will make sure that your visit is worth your time.

On the flip side, if your doctor is running a bit late (or really late) to an appointment, you need to be respectful enough to see that the waiting room is overflowing with patients and that your doctor is trying to care for everyone in the room, not just you. You also need to understand that running late is almost always beyond a doctor's control. For some insight into why, check out "A Typical Day in the Life of Your Doctor" below.

A TYPICAL DAY IN THE LIFE OF YOUR DOCTOR

I'm a regular guy. I wake up in the morning and get ready for work like most working people. I have breakfast, I interact with my family, I make plans for later in the day to spend time with my family and friends, and then I head to the office.

When I arrive at the office, I have a staff to check in with and share social niceties before I get down to business. There's a slew of messages for me to answer right away. The pharmacy has called to refill medications, and there are phone calls from patients who were admitted to the hospital overnight. All of these messages need my response, and all of this is happening before the first patient of the day has even arrived.

Once the patients start to arrive, there are still more fires to put out and people to deal with. A gastroenterologist calls about a patient with stomach problems that I referred to her, and we need to talk right now to formulate a plan. A patient in a nursing home has a fever, and I need to decide if they should be sent to the hospital. And all of this is happening while I'm seeing patients. There's also the matter of trying to get some nutrients into my body by way of eating lunch! I usually eat at my desk and use the time to catch up on charts or make phone calls. Pretty soon, I'm back at it.

Most doctors' schedules are set up to see patients every fifteen minutes—like clockwork. But this is assuming that the patients with diabetes, hypertension, heart failure, and high cholesterol are all problem-free for the day. (Which isn't very likely.) Patients with chronic diseases like these have great difficulty getting into the office and, once there, have many issues that need to be addressed. And then there's you, the patient, waiting patiently (or not so patiently) to be seen.

Patience, Patients, Please

Once you start to get an idea of what's going on in the mind of your doctor while they're trying to make time for you and trying to focus on you to make sure that you're happy at the end of your visit, you can understand that their limited time with you or the long wait isn't personal. The next time you're waiting around wondering when your name will be called, I hope you reflect on the responsibilities that your doctor is shouldering at that moment. And I hope that once your doctor does call you in, they say what I say to my patients that I've kept waiting, "I'm sorry."

I was seeing a patient once who was having crushing chest pain and had multiple risk factors like diabetes and hypertension. My waiting room was full, there was another patient whose fifteen minutes were fast approaching, but I needed to get this patient to an EKG machine. The test was abnormal, so then an ambulance had to be called to take this patient to the hospital to make sure that she wasn't having an acute heart attack. When the ambulance arrived, I had to speak with the ambulance staff and share my observances about how the patient presented and looked so we could all be on the same page as they moved forward with her care. And during all of this commotion, there was another patient in the other room waiting, getting angrier by the minute, without a clue about what was going on. She was going to be late for a job interview, and her doctor was nowhere to be found.

I learned two things from this experience:

1. No matter how crazy things are, I should always let the patient sitting in the other room know what's going on. Even if I can't get into specifics, it's enough to say, "We're having an emergency next door. I'll be with you soon." What the patient wants is for their doctor to acknowledge that they're there and that they've been waiting. That's usually enough to diffuse any tension. And if the doctor can't spare the time, then they should at least send in a nurse or a medical assistant. The absolute worst is when there's no communication. That's when a patient feels ignored and disrespected.

2. Having respect for someone means valuing their time as much as my own. It also means making things right with them, even when something wasn't technically my fault. So, in an instance like that, when I've unintentionally wasted a bunch of my patient's time, I give up my own time for them. I'll offer an appointment at a time or day that's best for them, even if it might not work for me. I've inconvenienced them (even if I didn't mean to) so I'll inconvenience myself.

Now, I realize that a lot of doctors don't necessarily do these two things, but I hope you still come away with the understanding that your doctor isn't intentionally disrespecting your time. Delays come with the nature of the business because, no matter how much we try to set a realistic schedule, a doctor's office isn't a factory that runs like clockwork.

Be on Time . . .

Given everything a doctor deals with in a day, there are so many things that can derail the train running on the fifteen-minute-slot track. Now what happens if a patient shows up twenty minutes late? Or worse, what if *two* patients are running behind? This directly impacts a doctor's ability to do all of these things outside of direct patient care in the office, along with getting home to be with their family. You might be thinking, *What about when my doctor is late in calling me in to be seen?* Well, it's most likely that a patient before you was late and threw off the schedule. And this is how tardiness can impact the entire day. It's a domino effect.

I've also heard this before: "I'm never seen on time so why should I be on time?" Now, living in New York City and knowing how public transportation can be, I always give my patients a grace period of ten minutes. And there can be some wiggle room in the schedule. But doctors are dealing with a lot of sick people each day. One late patient throws off the whole day, starting with their own visit. Plus, if you're seated on time, there's a chance you might be seen sooner. There's also plenty to do during the wait, including filling out medical forms. While you're waiting to be seen by your doctor, I recommend taking a few minutes to formulate your thoughts and, if you haven't done so already, write down a list of three things you want to have addressed in your visit. I know what it's like to leave the doctor's office and go, "Shoot, I wish I had asked about this problem!" So use your waiting time wisely to make sure that you make the most of your visit with your doctor.

Now, I'm going to say something that you, as a patient, might think is a little strange. Being "on time" to your appointment means arriving fifteen minutes early. Thirty minutes is even better, and forty-five minutes is a bonus. What's the benefit? Well, for one, you could potentially be seen sooner. If there's a patient who is a no-show and your name is on the list, you could take that person's time slot. But, if not, this additional time gives you a chance to get into the mind-set of focusing on your health and what you want to talk to your doctor about. You can fill out forms, take care of your copay and coinsurance, and speak with the office staff to address any administrative questions. You might be able to have your bloodwork done by the nurse before your time slot, giving the doctor a little extra time to spend with you. Plus, if you plan to arrive a half hour to forty-five minutes early, you can drive more leisurely and deal with any traffic or parking issues without worrying you will be late for your appointment.

With all that said, there are people who can't help but be chronically late. A patient may have an aid, and it takes a while to get to the office. In that case, I can't really fault them for being late. So my team and I decided that when we have patients who are relying on other people or services to get around and can't control their time management, we'll schedule them for the last appointment of the day. If the day ends at 5:00, we'll schedule them at 4:00, knowing that they'll likely arrive by 4:45 and we'll be able to give them the fifteen minutes they deserve.

Strategize When Making Your Appointment

Respect your doctor's time *and* your own by strategizing your appointment times. When you make an appointment, make sure there's some sort of plan around it. Don't just call the doctor's office and schedule the next available appointment.

Think about how your normal day usually works. Which is best for you? Mornings, afternoon, late afternoon, early evening? Do you have kids you need to pick up after school? If so, target early mornings. Do you need to see your doctor specifically during your lunch hour? Schedule your appointment for the start of your lunch hour, but make arrangements with your boss to make up any time missed the next day or later that day because there's no guarantee you'll be in and out within that window of time. Do you tend to rush around in the morning and will feel too stressed to make an appointment first thing in the morning? Pick an available appointment in the afternoon. Are certain days of the week busier for you than others? Choose a day when you have a lighter schedule.

Also, keep your other plans in mind. If you have another appointment that you *must* make on a certain day (like a job interview or hair appointment), avoid making an appointment that might potentially overlap with your other responsibilities. Or schedule your appointment for *after* that job interview or hair appointment. I realize that it can be challenging to get an appointment that works perfectly with your schedule, but at least have a plan of action before you arrive at the office.

Now I'm going to let you in on a little secret: One of the most effective times to see your doctor will likely be in the morning. That's when everyone's kind of bright-eyed and bushy-tailed and ready to go. Later in the day, we might be running behind (probably) and the glut of our day has caught up with us.

RESPECT OTHER PEOPLE'S EMERGENCIES

Let's say you have a 10:00 a.m. appointment, but the patient slotted for 9:45 needs more time with the doctor because it's an emergency situation that needs to be dealt with immediately. You feel put out and disrespected, but try to put yourself in the other person's shoes. Wouldn't you want extra time with the doctor if an emergency situation called for it? Every patient has a different idea of what an emergency means to them, so it's up to the doctor and staff to make that determination. We hope that you'll respect our ability to set patient priorities when necessary.

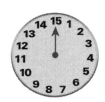

MAKING THE MOST OF YOUR 15 MINUTES

Fifteen minutes. That's generally all of the time your doctor has scheduled to see you. That's all of the time you have to speak your mind, feel heard, and find answers. That's not a lot of time! To make sure that patients and doctors make the most of their fifteen minutes together, I've put together a minute-by-minute breakdown of what an ideal visit looks like from your perspective as a patient.

MINUTES 1 and 2: The First Interaction

Your doctor greets you—warmly. Personally, I like to give my patients a handshake, grabbing them by the elbow or with two hands, to convey that I'm happy to see them, that this is going to be a good visit, that I'm going to try to make them better. Because physicians are people, too, and like to be greeted with a smile, if you're feeling well enough, offer your doctor a sincere smile. You can also ask your doctor how things are going; asking "How are you?" is a social nicety, but if you are very close with your doctor (which I hope you can be someday if you're not already), you can ask a more specific question, such as "How was your daughter's wedding last month?" or "How's that new grandson of yours?" or "How was your trip to Maui?" In general, we want to acknowledge each other as two people having an important interaction and make sure we start off on the right foot. Your doctor looks right at you (makes eye contact), not at the computer or the electronic medical record, to let you know that they are ready to see and hear you, really. You, too, look your doctor in the eye to let your doctor know that you are engaged and ready to focus on the problem or the issue that brought you there in in the first place.

MINUTES 3 and 4: Getting Settled

It's time to talk about you in general. To get the visit started, your doctor asks you how you've been since they last saw you. "How's life? What's been going on at home/work/school?" To make this question really count, be totally honest. This helps to set the tone and mood for the visit. You might say something along the lines of "It's great. Everything in my life has been going smoothly" or "I guess it could be better" or "I'm having problems at work" or "I'm struggling in a class" and so on. Your doctor considers your chief complaint (why is this patient here?) and considers if your answers to these questions have any bearing on your current state of health. So be very, very honest with your answers.

MINUTES 5, 6, and 7:
The Heart of the Matter

Your doctor asks what brings you in today. When you made the appointment, you likely told the staff why you needed to see the doctor, and so your doctor knows what your chief complaint is; however, they need to hear it directly from you. When you are the only one talking, that minute or so is going to feel like a lot of time. Use it up. If you say, "I have a nagging cough" for instance, you have time to offer more information about it: "I've had a nagging cough for two weeks. I had a cold a few weeks ago, but I didn't start coughing until after it went away. It's a very dry cough. I don't feel it in my chest; it's more in my throat. It's worse at night, and it's interfering with my sleep. I've tried cough medicines and they help a little, but it's just not going away. I've also been getting headaches. Mostly in the morning. I don't know if it's connected or anything, but I thought it's important to mention."

As you are speaking, your doctor listens to you speak, *really* listens. Your doctor makes you feel heard and comfortable by using nonverbal and verbal cues, like nodding, facial expressions, and simple phrases like "Yes," "Uh huh," and "I understand." Your doctor may ask a question or two for clarification, and as you respond as fully as possible, your doctor keeps listening and doesn't interrupt.

MINUTES 8 and 9:
The Examination and Questions

During the examination, your doctor treats you like an important individual who has come to them for help rather than just another patient to service and get out of there. You don't have to do anything during this time except listen for your doctor's prompts and commands such as "lie back" and "breathe deeply." Your doctor will also ask questions to get a better idea of what's going on, such as "Where does the pain radiate?" or Does the pain move around?" or "Does it hurt when I press here?" Your doctor will ask additional questions regarding your symptoms to get a fuller picture of your complaint. For instance, your doctor might ask, "What makes you feel better?" In other words, is there anything you do that you've noticed that alleviates your symptoms at least for a while. And "What makes it worse?" In other words, have you noticed anything in particular that triggers your symptoms or makes them more severe?

MINUTE 10:
The Diagnosis

You doctor puts a name to what you've been experiencing, and hopefully you find comfort. It's possible that further tests will be required to ascertain what is causing your symptoms. In that case, your doctor will tell you which tests are being ordered and what those tests are looking for. If your doctor determines that your condition can be improved or your health can be maintained with certain medication, they will talk about that now.

MINUTE 11:
Medication Reconciliation

Your doctor will go through a medication reconciliation process, reviewing any medications on your record to see if you are still taking that medication, if you are doing okay with that medication, and so on. You might be what we doctors lovingly refer to as an "invincible"—a relatively young and healthy patient who isn't on any medication. That's great! This means there's more time for other aspects of your office visit.

MINUTE 12:
Preventative Care Reminders

Your doctor will let you know if you're due for any "routine maintenance." Have you had your mammogram, your pap smear, colonoscopy, etc.?

MINUTE 13:
Review of Past Appointments

Your doctor will review any past problems you've addressed at previous appointments to determine if your current concerns and symptoms are related to any prior issues.

MINUTE 14:
Patient Education

Your doctor now takes time to educate you about what you've discussed at your appointment. This is when I pull out my handy dry erase board and exercise my "artistic talent." Maybe your pain is related to gallstones, and you want to know more about your gallbladder. Now is a good time to ask for clarification if anything is confusing to you about your particular condition or about anything your doctor is recommending.

MINUTE 15:
Your Good-byes

It's time to part ways. Your doctor thanks you for coming in and trusting them with your care. You thank your doctor for taking the time to see you and address your concerns. You reiterate what you heard your doctor tell you with regard to your next steps so that your doctor knows you fully understand their recommendations or can correct you if necessary.

Also, think about whether or not you've brought up everything you wanted your doctor to know or ask any questions you'd forgotten to ask. Although this is a bit of a hyperbole, there's nothing worse than leaving the doctor's office and having someone ask you later on, "Why did your doctor say about such and such?" And you have to reply that you forgot to ask. So, as you are wrapping up the appointment, try to think about some things that weren't necessarily addressed or that you want to talk about on your follow-up visit. This can be a little bit challenging for doctors because our visit with you is winding down, but that's okay. It at least allows us to say, "Okay, we didn't get a chance to talk about that. Let's figure out our next appointment. Or I can give you a call back and talk to you about that" or "I'll send in the nurse to answer that."

Now, ideally, at the end of your doctor's visit, you feel happy, fulfilled, and respected. You leave knowing that you were truly heard and that your time was well spent. If not? Then I encourage you to go over this fifteen-minute breakdown and figure out where things went awry. What did or didn't happen that might be impacting your relationship?

◀ BEHIND THE CURTAIN ▶

A while back, I was working at a practice in the Beverly Hills area, and I had a patient who would come in fairly often, but we weren't really developing that close bond I want to have with my patients. In a roundabout way, he had intimated that because he lived outside LA in an area he didn't seem proud of, he wasn't as valued as my other patients who were residents of Beverly Hills. I could tell this made him reticent to share with me, but I never pushed the discussion because he hadn't really said anything outright to me about this.

Then, at one appointment, I noticed something particularly off about his demeanor. When I pressed a bit, he admitted that there were some things going on, but then said bluntly and maybe a little condescendingly, "You wouldn't understand, Dr. Redcross."

I kind of chuckled a bit to myself and asked, "What would you mean by that?"

He replied, "Look at you, here you are in the middle of Beverly Hills. You're young and you have everything. Your patients have everything, too. I can't even imagine how you could understand what I'm going through, or even what I've been through in life."

"Try me," I said.

He explained how rough his upbringing had been and how certain people continue to make his life even more of a challenge. He had relatives relying on him for support and children who weren't making good decisions.

I sat down and said, "Let me tell you a little bit about my story. This isn't to compare myself to you, but I just want you to know where I'm coming from."

I explained to him that I was born into modest means. "My parents were beautiful, hardworking people, but I didn't have any role models in medicine to suggest I could actually go on to become a physician someday. Eventually, I became the first physician in my family, but it didn't happen without challenges."

I went on to tell him how, in the nineties, I took a position in the ER at a hospital in Harlem, New York. The area was pretty rough back then, but I felt comfortable, needed, and loved among people I knew needed me (some of whom actually checked into the ER just to get out of the cold). I felt very much at home and as if I was supposed to be there making a difference.

Yes, the train rides home were dangerous, but it was all worth it to me, to be able to make a difference at that hospital. I also told my patient that I could relate to relatives who weren't doing what I want them to do and that I understood tragedies close to home and what it means to have to pick up pieces.

"Hey, look," I said, "this may be where I am, but this isn't how I define myself or anyone else. At the end of the day, I think people are people and healing transcends any kind of background, ethnicity, community, or location."

"Gosh, I didn't know you were able to roll like that," he said, half-jokingly.

For me and this patient, this conversation was a really big breakthrough. I had gained his respect by sharing a little about myself, and he opened up more fully, and I was really able to help him. This helped me, too, because up until that point, I hadn't really thought much about how all my past experiences had molded me into the physician I am today.

Respecting Your Doctor's Decisions

It might work in the dressing room, but in medicine, one size *does not* fit all. Every single patient and every single situation is different, so a doctor needs to consider a variety of factors before arriving at a decision and then needs to communicate to the patient, "I'm making this decision for *you* because . . ." If there are options for the patient to choose from, that needs to be mentioned as well.

Patients need to remember that they are unique, and what might be true for a family member or friend won't necessarily be true for them. You might say, "Well, you know, doc, I have a friend with diabetes and her doctor said she doesn't need any pills right now, so why do I?" Your doctor doesn't know your friend's medical history and what factors went into her doctor's decision. There's nothing wrong with comparing and contrasting, but your doctor can only do for you what your particular history and current condition suggest is necessary.

Questioning every recommendation your doctor makes for you borders on disrespectful. This isn't the same thing as asking, "Is it really necessary for me to take this medication?" That's a valid question. Your doctor may say that it is absolutely necessary to get you better or keep you balanced, but they may also offer you options or take your preferences into consideration. But no matter the case, respect that your doctor has your best interests at heart when making recommendations.

Sometimes, doctors need to respect their patient's wishes, too. This is especially true when it comes to religious beliefs. For instance, if a patient is anemic and requires a blood transfusion but, for religious reasons, will not have this procedure (as would be the case with Jehovah's Witnesses), I can have a serious discussion with the patient about why I think it's necessary, but ultimately, I have to respect that person's beliefs.

In other cases, a patient may want to try homeopathic or natural remedies rather than the medication I am prescribing. I respect people who want to avoid taking medication if it's not absolutely necessary, and if there's a natural remedy that can cure their condition or ease their symptoms that they want to try, I'm all for it. However, I need these patients to respect my training and education enough to take me seriously when I say, "The standard of care, the best practices show that you're going to need a prescription for this to get well or stay healthy." I hope that my patient will then turn around and say, "All right, in my case, Dr. Redcross has told me why he believes I need to take this, and I'm going to respect his decision."

CULTIVATING RESPECT CHEAT SHEET

✓ If you're seeing a new doctor, start with a clean slate. Consciously set aside old experiences or assumptions that might cloud your impressions of your new physician and approach them with the intention of forming a mutually respectful relationship.

✓ Always show up to your appointment on time. (Fifteen minutes early is on time.) Showing up late may mean the patients who come after you will have their appointments delayed as a result. Everyone's time is of equal importance.

✓ Write down three things that you want to talk to your doctor about before your visit. This will help you make the most of your visit.

✓ Be patient when your doctor is running behind. Your doctor's desire to help you get better extends to every one of their patients, and they're making sure each patient—yourself included—is getting the right amount of attention and care.

✓ Recognize that your doctor's primary goal is to help you get better, and respect that everything they advise you to do comes from that desire. Be open to hearing what they have to say.

✓ Always answer your doctor's questions honestly. If your doctor asks how you're doing, they're asking not only because they're interested in getting to know you but because your answer might provide them the insight to help you resolve your chief complaint.

✓ Remember that what works for a friend or family member may not work for you. If your doctor prescribes something different from what you were expecting, understand that they're doing so because you and your situation are unique. Your doctor can only judge what's happening with you, not with your peers. Expect that your doctor has your personal best interests at heart.

✓ If you're uncertain about treatment options or other aspects of your diagnosis, ask questions. Your doctor should not be dismissive of your concerns, nor should you be embarrassed if you don't fully understand their advice. Reiterate their advice to make sure you're both on the same page.

✓ If you don't feel happy, fulfilled, or respected by the end of your visit, mentally review the visit and try to identify where things went wrong.

From Doctor to Doctor

Here are some approaches that have worked for me in my practice to help deepen the level of respect between my patients and me. Maybe you will find them helpful as well for cultivating respect and solidifying the patient-doctor bond you have with your patients.

- I always take an interest in my patients' profession or hobbies. I recognize that these aspects of my patients' lives are no less valuable or important than my own.

- I use the fifteen-minute guide to make the most of every visit to be sure to give my patient enough time to express themselves fully.

- During our time together, I treat each patient like my primary priority and give them my full attention. I set aside whatever happened previously and what I still have to accomplish that day. In other words, I practice being fully in the moment.

- If I'm running behind schedule, I make sure that my staff keeps my patients in the loop. Too often, a patient will be waiting in a doctor's waiting room and the time keeps ticking by and they have no idea when they will be called, which causes frustration. So when they check in, I make sure that a member of my staff lets them know approximately how long they can expect to wait. If there's an emergency that's keeping me occupied for a longer time, I make sure my staff informs the patients in the waiting room.

- When I've made a patient wait, I apologize. I realize that this isn't always in my control, but I am able to control how I respond to a patient's complaints about the wait.

CHAPTER 5

Empathy: Seeing Each Other from a Common Perspective

"The patient will never care how much you know, until they know how much you care."

—Dr. Terry Canale

When a patient comes to my office, I want them to understand that I'm here to *heal* them—not just write a prescription. Healing for me means figuring out why my patient is having certain symptoms—is it stress, anxiety, diet, something else? I need to help my patient heal on that level so that they can make better decisions going forward. I want them to know that I am coming from a place of true concern; I want them to *understand* me and my motivations. But I can't do this without first listening to them with an empathetic ear. That means not jumping to conclusions based on the symptoms they present and withholding judgment until I've heard the whole story. It means seeing them as individuals and not comparing them to my other patients, although my experience with other patients is valuable information. It means trying to understand their unique perspective and experiences.

In the *7 Habits of Highly Effective People,* Stephen Covey reminds us of what I live by as a doctor: "Diagnose Before You Prescribe." He discusses the importance of empathetic listening within Habit 5: Seek First to Understand, Then to Be Understood,[20] and I believe this goes for both patients and doctors, as I'll discuss throughout this chapter. Hopefully, we can come out on the other side with a good understanding of how this cornerstone quality is one we should all strive to establish in our doctor-patient relationship because, without it, we're missing an essential factor in the human equation.

Empathy: Healthcare's Hot-Button Topic

In healthcare today, the focus has been on the need for doctors to be more empathetic with their patients. I'll get into how empathy is a two-way street in any relationship later, but for now, let's look at the doctor's side of the equation. Gone are the days when it was believed that doctors needed to erect emotional barriers to keep from becoming overwhelmed by their patients' problems. It is entirely possible to empathize with another person without becoming so emotionally invested in them that we take on their feelings and problems as our own. That's codependency, not empathy.

Empathy, the ability to understand what another person is feeling, is essential in a lasting and caring patient-doctor relationship. In fact, empathy can be key to medical efficacy. A 2018 article in *The Atlantic* cites a study showing that the rate of severe diabetes complications in patients of doctors who rate high on a standard empathy scale is 40 percent lower than in patients with low-empathy doctors.[21] Diabetes is one of those disease states where the patient may feel 100 percent fine, but to prevent severe complications, the patient must be diligent about keeping their hemoglobin A1C levels in check. It's hard to get through to these patients, especially young ones, who don't want to have to deal with diabetes or face the stigma of having to carry around needles and/or take pills in front of their peers. Doctors who are able to empathize with these patients have a better chance of getting through to them than doctors who throw their hands up in the air in frustration and say, "Well, I told you, and now it's up to you." A more emphatic response would be, "You know, I understand how it is to be twenty, and I understand how it is to want to go out with your friends and not have to inject yourself or take pills. I know it's not easy, but to keep you healthy, we are going to have to figure this out together."

To establish a strong bond in any relationship, we must have empathy for one another. A doctor needs to consider their patient's perspective to fully grasp their fears, concerns, desires, etc., with regard to their health. When a doctor is able to do this, the patient feels like the doctor truly cares—like they have someone by their side who's going through the trenches with them. But a doctor can't empathize with their patients unless they understand what's really going through their patients' minds and what they're dealing with—and they can't know this unless the patient is forthcoming and the doctor listens carefully to that patient when they speak.

That's why empathy cannot exist without communication, respect, and trust. It's important that you trust and respect your doctor enough to communicate with them exactly what you are experiencing, and I don't just mean that you tell your doctor that you're having chest pains but how those chest pains make you feel: frightened, concerned, worried, or whatever it is that those chest pains are making you feel on a deeper level than just physically. This gives your doctor the chance to say, "I understand that you're frightened. We're going to get through it together."

When you tell your doctor that your dad died of a heart attack, for instance, and you're afraid that you're headed down the same path, it gives the doctor an opportunity to bring in their own personal experiences as well. Maybe they've lost a parent to heart disease, too. "I know how it feels to lose a parent to that disease. Fortunately, we know more than they did back then, and we'll get to the root of the problem using today's modern medicine."

When a doctor lets down their shield, they become more relatable to their patients, and that's how we build a strong connection—by being a little vulnerable on both sides during our interactions. Being vulnerable can be unnerving to a doctor. I love to get personal, but I know that not every doctor is wired that way. So perhaps your doctor doesn't want to share personal anecdotes to relate to you; they may have a different way of showing you that they care. As a patient, I want you to know that it's "daring" for your doctor to care, but also that it's a critical quality to cultivate and it's easier than a doctor might think. A recent survey found that many doctors struggle with the feeling that they're spending more time taking notes than talking to a patient, and even more with the feeling that the patient thinks so, too. Physicians feel they're being under-utilized in their profession because oversight demands they spend so much time checking boxes that they never really get to connect with their patients.[22] This is a real challenge, one that doctors need to deal with on a daily basis. Fortunately, it is possible to express empathy in the fifteen minutes allotted to the visit when the intention is sincere.

◀ BEHIND THE CURTAIN ▶

One of my elderly patients lives in a primary care facility. She has four children, but one daughter is her primary caretaker. This daughter has devoted eight years of her life to tending to her mother, and she's had to do it all by herself. Sometimes, her brother and sisters will come to visit, but when they do, it's mostly to criticize. "I went to see Mom, and it looks like no one is tending to her," they'll say to their sister accusingly. "She's not being fed and bathed the way she should. Are you taking care of her finances?" This criticism only adds to her burden. Her mother is now ninety years old and getting ill, and she's beginning to realize that her mother likely won't be around much longer. This thought gives her some relief. Her mother will pass without too much suffering, and things will be easier. This thought also brings her an enormous amount of guilt. Yes, she's had to put her life on hold, but she can barely admit to anyone—including herself—that she wants to start living again.

We talk very openly about her conflicted feelings. She asks me, "Am I such a bad person? My mother is so wonderful, but I'm tired. I'm just ready to turn the page." She feels awful. And I empathize with how she feels. She thinks she's alone in this. She thinks that no one else understands. But what she doesn't know is that this is such a common situation. I hear it every day. I hear the fear and the frustration and the isolation.

I also hear the kindness and the selflessness. This woman had wanted to go back to school and further her career. She wanted to start a family. But she dropped all of that to be there for her mother. She made a major sacrifice, and she wasn't giving herself enough credit. She was in such a fog, thinking that she was just doing what she was supposed to do, and she couldn't see her actions for what they were: acts of heroism. So instead of focusing on her guilt, we talk about that. We talk about her goodness. I tell her about my experiences with my own parents. I tell her that I know what she wishes she could say to her siblings: *Why don't you fill out the forms? Why don't you make the appointments?* I tell her that I get it. I get her. I get that she has guilt that's trapped inside her heart and soul. And maybe what I tell her isn't enough to release that guilt. But knowing that someone else understands how she feels is enough to help her keep going.

Getting to Know You

When we're invested in a relationship, we show that we care by asking questions about the other person's life. We want to know what their hobbies are, the types of experiences they had as children, what their family life is like, who their favorite sports team are, and so on. I realize there's not a lot of time during those fifteen minutes when you are meeting with your doctor, but it's great when you and your doctor can engage each other in these types of conversations, no matter how brief, to get to know each other on a human level.

One of my favorite things to talk about with patients is family. I'm an only child and don't know what it's like to be close to a sibling, so I especially love hearing about people's brothers and sisters. I've also learned that so many people are proud of their parents, and it can be really powerful to hear why. Other times, I'll talk to patients who've had rough upbringings, and I'm moved by their stories. One of my patients is a business executive, and when I asked if her parents are proud of her, she said, "Eh, my parents were sort of hippies, so everything was loosey-goosey in my house. They did their own thing. They weren't really involved." That was a tough thing to hear, but I'm grateful I was able to learn about her background because it helped me better understand her as a person and made our bond stronger. It also gave me the chance to tell her, as I tell all of my patients who've faced challenges in their life, that I think she's an absolute warrior.

Another question I always make a point of asking is "What's your dream? Maybe you're an accountant right now, but what would you be doing if you could do anything you wanted?" Immediately, my patients start smiling because that thought excites them. And then, when they inevitably come back down to earth and tell me, "Oh, but I don't have the money," or "I'm just not smart or talented enough," I say, "Hold on, pump the breaks. What can we do to make that dream a reality?" I love to dream chase like that!

A registered nurse once came to see me, and she told me that she had always wanted to go to medical school but never did. When I asked why she didn't consider that now, she responded that she just really loves nursing. But I told her not to give up on her goal of higher education. Over the years, we built a bond, and she did end up going after her dreams. She's now a nurse practitioner with an MBA, and my heart is full just thinking that I played even half a percent in helping her get there.

I have just two rules that I follow when it comes to asking my patients about themselves:

1. If my patient tells me that they "hate" something, I help them turn it around so that they can focus on positive aspects and ways they can make a change.

2. No topic is too personal, unless my patient says so.

Your doctor might not ask you questions like this, but it's probably not because they don't care about you as a person and wouldn't be interested in learning more about you. You can offer this type of information and potentially get your doctor to open up about themselves, too. This is how we bring our humanity into the patient-doctor relationship.

◀ BEHIND THE CURTAIN ▶

Years back, I worked in a methadone clinic, helping in the recovery of those who were saddled with addiction. It's unfortunate, but much of our society has a preconceived notion that people in a drug addiction program are weak and morally afflicted. Before I took the position, I was inclined to believe that they were in these programs because they had done something wrong or were at fault. Even with my early prejudices, I realized that there was a lot more to this than I knew, and I wanted to hear their stories. But, truthfully, I went into this thinking I might be hearing a bunch of woe-is-me tales.

Early on, one patient changed my way of trying to lump a multitude of various life experiences into some sort of "hard knocks" category. This patient had been born into and had grown up in a drug-infested house; she didn't know any other way of life. As I listened to her story, I tried to put myself in her place. I wondered if I would have survived as well as she had, here in her thirties and voluntarily entered into a methadone program. How would I have been able to navigate those waters? The more I learned about her, the more impressed I became. She had a goal to become financially independent and had created a revenue-generating business from legally acquiring items left behind in abandoned apartments and selling them. She was so appreciative that I had taken an interest in her, but that day, I was the grateful one. I recognized that while we shared an entrepreneurial spirt, she had many more challenges to contend with to achieve success than I did. I was able to tell her in all honesty, "As far as I'm concerned, you are a hero, and I know you can do this because you have already done so much." A lot of other people in these programs are heroes as well in their efforts to battle addiction.

Through hearing her story and those of others, I quickly realized that I had been so far off base with my thinking of how people come to these facilities. By the time I completed my service at the clinic, I had a better understanding of what it means to walk a mile in someone's shoes: We can't possibly judge another without taking time to try to understand their perspectives and experiences.

We're All Human

To understand one another, we must first recognize each other's humanity. I've worked all over the country, from Beverly Hills to Harlem, and at the end of the day, no matter where you go, patients are patients, doctors are doctors, and we're all just human beings.

For a patient to recognize a doctor's humanity, I think it's important for doctors to open up, be vulnerable, and admit mistakes. Personally, I share experiences about what I've been through or about my family just to say look, "I'm here with you. I know how that felt for me. I hear where you are coming from." It takes a patient from being with the doctor in this cold room down to a friend or family member who's in your living room with the purpose of supporting you and making you feel better. Not every doctor has to do that; some don't feel comfortable, and I get that. But when a patient has dealt with something traumatic like losing a child in late-term pregnancy, and several emotions are rising to the surface, it's important to let her into my soul for the moment to say: "I've been there. You're not alone. I can imagine how you feel, and I know that you can pick up the pieces and go through life. You will be able to do it, and this will make you an even stronger person." I don't have to share a story like that with my patient, no doctor does, and patients know that. That's what makes it so special and so powerful. It takes down the guard between the doctor and the patient so that we can understand each other on common ground.

Sometimes, though, the act of empathy involves simply listening without offering my own personal experiences. I know there are certain experiences I could never fully understand without having experienced it myself, so I walk the fine line between trying to relate and knowing when all I need to do is listen.

Another way I allow myself to show my humanity is to own a mistake. I admit it and try to make things right. Maybe I wasn't as engaged as I should have been with a patient. That patient calls me out: "Look, you weren't paying attention. I wanted more time." Instead of saying that's just the way it is, I try to see things from their point of view. Whether I agree with what they're saying or not, they're telling me what they perceive, and I have to acknowledge that. I have to apologize. I have to be humble. Not just because I think it's the right thing to do, but because it shows that I'm human, too.

Expressing Gratitude for Each Other

Gratitude is the way we show someone that we appreciate and understand the time and attention they have given us. A simple thank you goes a long way toward recognizing someone's efforts to help you or make your life a little easier in some way, even if it is as simple as holding open a door. The expression of gratitude between patient and doctor goes both ways. It's certainly not uncommon for a patient and doctor to share the social nicety "thank you" in parting, but expressing gratitude can be taken to another, deeper level. For example, when a new patient joins my practice, I send them a thank-you card. They could have picked any doctor, and they picked me—trusted me—to care for them. It may seem like such a small thing, but I believe that there are few things more powerful than a card when you want to express gratitude.

WELCOME TO THE REDCROSS CONCIERGE FAMILY!

We are thrilled to offer you member services Dr. Ken Redcross believes everyone deserves: comprehensive care focusing on not only your physical body, but your soul and spirit as well. Thank you for trusting us with your care as we ensure preventative and holistic treatment, medical counsel, education, and personalized custom care.

WELCOME TO THE KIND OF CARE THAT ALWAYS PUTS YOU AT THE FOREFRONT OF WELLNESS. WE LOOK FORWARD TO A HEALTHY RELATIONSHIP!

Dr. Ken Redcross

THANK YOU

REDCROSS CONCIERGE

Dr. Ken's New Patient Thank-You Card

Do you have any idea how much something as simple as a thank-you card can enhance your relationship with your doctor? It will likely be the highlight of their day. Why? Because unfortunately, it almost never happens. And it's not because patients aren't appreciative of their physicians. It's because they can't help but take for granted that it's their job to fix them. But like you, your doctor feels good when they're thanked or praised for a job well done.

If you want to really show your appreciation, you can grab a thank-you card and put pen to paper. That melts my heart. And that's for two reasons: One, I never expect anyone to thank me for doing what I love to do. And, two, I'm so touched by the notion that the patient actually thought about me outside of the office and went to the trouble of getting a card and writing words in it. And heartfelt words at that. That sort of thing has always reinforced what I do.

◀ BEHIND THE CURTAIN ▶

I had just transitioned from my residency in New York to California, and I was thoroughly overwhelmed. I was at a new clinic as a new attending, trying to fit in while also wanting to make my mark. I was winging it. And all the while, I was drowning a little bit, 3,000 thousand miles from home.

On a particularly stressful day after seeing approximately thirty patients, I was feeling a little lost. I remember thinking, *I know this is what it means to be a doctor, but it's not speaking to me right now.* It was early in my career, and I was still learning who I was as a doctor and what I loved about my profession. I needed something, but I wasn't sure what.

Just then, a new patient walked through the door. It was a nun—a full-fledged nun—habit and all. I mean, can you believe it? I was having a rough day, starting to question everything, hoping for a sign from above, and suddenly there's a nun in my waiting room!

After that first meeting, Sister Beatrice and I became very close. She would invite me down to the convent, where I would spend time with her and her sisters on the weekend. We would speak about spirituality, and I started to feel whole again thanks to our connection.

One day, she told me that she was about to go on a mission and wouldn't be coming back. I was heartbroken but also grateful for the time we had together. She said she wanted to give me something to thank me and to remember her by. She handed me a small silver cross that opened up like a locket. I held it in my hands in awe. It was a precious gift.

Ever since that day, I've carried around that cross like a talisman. It was a gift from a beloved patient, but it was also so much more—it was a constant reminder. It reminded me of how blessed I was. It reminded me of what I'm called to do as a doctor. It reminded me that I could battle all things that come my way. It reminded me of that day, that pivotal moment that molded me over the next seventeen years, that taught me the power of the patient-doctor bond.

I'll never forget Sister Beatrice, just as I'll never forget my purpose.

Bringing Back the House Call

In my opinion, one of the best ways doctors can show their patients that they are there for them is with a house call. In the 1960s, house calls by doctors were 40 percent of patient-doctor meetings. By 1980, they were only 0.6 percent.[23] There are many reasons why the frequency of house calls has gone down so dramatically: for one, many doctors need to see far too many patients in one day to be able to take the time out of their schedule to visit a single patient (remember, "A Typical Day in the Life of Your Doctor" on page 64?). Also, in the case of some patients and illnesses, it's important to have the support staff at the ready to be able to run tests or perform other necessary functions.[24] With that said, I will still argue that the house call resurrects what is sorely missing in health-care today.

When a doctor makes a house call to a patient, they create a foundation for something beautiful to be hoisted up for years to come—they have a patient for life. The patient feels that they're important enough to be seen on their turf. The doctor is also able to learn about them by experiencing their environment and the challenges they may face. Once a doctor enters a patient's world, they can discover so much that they wouldn't have otherwise known. For example, I have a patient who is very spiritual, and when I was making a house call, I discovered that she had a meditation area. This gave me so much insight into how she manages her stress and sort of opened a window into who she is as a person. During an office visit, I would never have asked, "So, do you have a meditation room?" I would have never known that. Instead, I mentioned that I also meditate and we discovered that we had a similar approach to dealing with life, and it brought us closer. That's the power of the house call.

One of the greatest benefits of the house call is how utterly personal the experience can be for the patient and the doctor. There's no sitting in a waiting room with a dozen other sick people. Instead, the patient feels they can be more open and honest with their doctor. There's nothing to hide. Going directly to the patient helps them feel like they're important, unique, and worthy of a doctor's time, energy, and personalized concern. The doctor, in turn, feels like they're getting to know their patient better. This mutual feeling of comfort allows both doctor and patient to open up to one another, and empathy grows in that space.

FOSTERING EMPATHY CHEAT SHEET

✓ Open up about your life. What are your interests? What are your challenges? Getting to know you as a person will help your doctor to empathize with you. If they don't know what's going on in your mind, they can't bond with you. Opening up to your doctor from the get-go will also help your doctor recognize when something in your mood or behavior changes, so they can identify if such changes point to a change in your overall health.

✓ Dare to share your dreams with your doctor. They may provide you with the motivation to go for it.

✓ Are you grateful for your doctor? Tell them! A simple thank-you, verbal or written, shows you appreciate your doctor's concern for you and you recognize that their goal, first and foremost, is to help you get and stay healthy.

✓ Be aware that not everyone is comfortable being vulnerable. If your doctor is a little hesitant to be open about their personal life, it's not because they don't want to bond with you. They just might show their feelings differently.

✓ If you feel you're not being heard or your doctor has made a mistake, approach the situation with the knowledge that we're all human and we all make mistakes. Try to be as understanding as possible. But do tell your doctor politely and honestly so they can remedy the situation. Keeping such concerns to yourself can put a wedge between you and your doctor that may prevent you from getting the best possible care—and the best possible care is your doctor's primary goal.

From Doctor to Doctor

Here are some approaches that have worked for me in my practice to help deepen this cornerstone between my patients and me. Maybe you will find them helpful as well for fostering empathy and solidifying the patient-doctor bond you have with your patients.

- My patients always appreciate when I give them a phone call to check in. My approach to making calls to my patients is kind of organic and spiritual. If I'm at home or in the office and I start thinking of a patient, I will pick up the phone or text that patient. I usually make it a point to check in with patients who have had a procedure to see how they're doing or if I know that a certain patient is grappling with a serious challenge. I have tailored my practice so that I can deliver this sort of attention to my patients, and I realize that this isn't the case with large practices. But even calling two patients a month can make a huge difference, which could have a ripple effect, making everyone it touches feel awesome and special.

- During an office visit, I engage my patients by asking about their lives. What's their family like? What's their dream? And I share personal stories that relate to my patients' experiences, which deepens our bond and connection.

- I always apologize when I haven't kept a promise to a patient or when I'm unable to meet a patient's expectations. For instance, if I promised a patient a phone call and I got so busy that I forgot all about it, I will call that patient at the next opportunity to say I'm sorry—even if it's a couple of days later when I remember.

■ We physicians have a lot on our minds—not just about work but about our regular lives, too. We're also trying our best to keep up with patients during visits, while inputting electronic data, all the while thinking of their diagnosis or treatment. These responsibilities can make us feel the need to withdraw emotionally from our patients in order to be efficient. On a particular day if I think that my need to be efficient may override my ability to connect with my patients as human beings, I stop myself and dare to care. I make the small gestures with big impact, knowing that I still need to go the extra mile to show that I'm there for my patients no matter the responsibilities that are weighing on me that day.

■ In all honestly, not every one of my patients is easy to like (and not everyone is going to like me!). I try to have empathy for these people, too, no matter how sour they may be toward me. I don't blame the patient for not being a joy; instead I try to figure out how to make the visit joyful anyway, using humor if appropriate, but always kindness. Although the interaction might not be what my patient and I would like it to be, I don't let this ruin the rest of my day or spill into my time with the next patient. The common sports phrase "leave it all on the field" comes into play here for me. While I'm "playing," I give it all I've got, and no matter the outcome, I know I did my best. I always end the interaction with "I look forward to our next visit." Even if that's a bit of a stretch, I hope it will be the opening we need for a better interaction next time.

CHAPTER 6

Time to Assess:
Filling Out the Patient-Doctor Relationship Evaluation

At this point, you should have a good idea of my perspective on the four cornerstones of the patient-doctor bond and what a healthy relationship between patients and doctors looks like. The only question left is: How's *your* relationship with *your* doctor?

Only you can answer that question. I can't tell you how happy and healthy you are. But I do want to help. That's why I've put together a guide for how to evaluate the strength of your patient-doctor bond. In this chapter, you'll find a "relationship report card" that you can use to grade your unique bond with your doctor. After scoring the results, you'll be able to determine for yourself if (and how much) your relationship needs improvement. We'll also discuss whether or not you should consider breaking up with your doctor and how best to do this.

The Patient-Doctor Relationship Evaluation

Keeping in mind everything you've read in the previous chapters, take some time to consider each of the prompts below before you answer. Be as honest with yourself as possible as you answer them because how you respond will affect how you proceed hereafter, in terms of your personal health. Rate each question on a scale from 1 to 5, and tally the subtotal after each section. When you're done evaluating each of the four cornerstone qualities, combine all four subtotals to get your final score.

TRUST

	Strongly Disagree	Disagree	Neutral	Agree	Strongly Agree
I feel that I can tell my doctor anything.	1	2	3	4	5
I feel that my doctor's office is a no-judgment zone.	1	2	3	4	5
I feel like I have my guard down when I'm with my doctor.	1	2	3	4	5
I believe that my doctor is always honest with me.	1	2	3	4	5
	Never	Rarely	Sometimes	Often	Always
My doctor takes times to educate and explain things to me.	1	2	3	4	5
My doctor is open to hearing about research I've done on my own.	1	2	3	4	5

SUBTOTAL:_____

COMMUNICATION

	Strongly Disagree	Disagree	Neutral	Agree	Strongly Agree
I feel that my doctor really hears me when I speak.	1	2	3	4	5
I feel that I can ask my doctor anything.	1	2	3	4	5
I feel comfortable giving my doctor feedback.	1	2	3	4	5

Communication (cont.)

	Never	Rarely	Sometimes	Often	Always
My doctor explains things to me in ways that I understand.	1	2	3	4	5
My doctor follows up with test results in a timely manner.	1	2	3	4	5
My doctor is able to address all of the concerns that I have.	1	2	3	4	5
				SUBTOTAL:	

RESPECT

	Strongly Disagree	Disagree	Neutral	Agree	Strongly Agree
I feel that my time is well spent after seeing my doctor.	1	2	3	4	5
I feel that my doctor treats me like a person and not an appointment.	1	2	3	4	5
I never feel demeaned or belittled by my doctor.	1	2	3	4	5
	Never	Rarely	Sometimes	Often	Always
My doctor takes an interest in what I do for a living.	1	2	3	4	5
My doctor apologizes when I have to wait for a while.	1	2	3	4	5
My doctor listens to me when I speak (without interrupting).	1	2	3	4	5
				SUBTOTAL:	

EMPATHY					
	Strongly Disagree	Disagree	Neutral	Agree	Strongly Agree
I feel like my doctor and I are in this together.	1	2	3	4	5
I feel like my doctor makes an effort to go the extra mile.	1	2	3	4	5
	Never	Rarely	Sometimes	Often	Always
My doctor asks questions about my life.	1	2	3	4	5
My doctor shows gratitude for having me as a patient.	1	2	3	4	5
My doctor acts genuinely happy to see me.	1	2	3	4	5
My doctor shows their human side.	1	2	3	4	5
				SUBTOTAL:_____	

TRUST _____

+ COMMUNICATION _____

+ RESPECT _____

+ EMPATHY _____

= TOTAL _____

SCORING:

96–120 Points—Congratulations! It seems like you have a strong bond with your doctor. My advice to you: Cherish it and tend to it as it grows. After all, relationships aren't static; they're dynamic, living things. Use this book as a guide for how to strengthen your patient-doctor bond as it changes and keep it healthy over the years. And, if you're really happy with your doctor, let them know! Take your relationship to the next level by writing your doctor a thoughtful thank-you note.

49–95 Points—Your relationship with your doctor could use some work. Luckily, you have all the tools you need to fix it right in your hands. Start by evaluating your subtotals to determine which qualities need the most attention. Then go back and review the associated chapters in this book for advice on how to strengthen your bond with your doctor—and get even closer to reaching "patient nirvana."

0–48 Points—Your relationship with your doctor could use a lot of improvement. While it may seem like a daunting task, you can start by pinpointing the three weakest areas and making those your top priorities. The patient-doctor bond is a lengthy and ever-evolving journey, but it begins with a series of small, focused steps. If you're not making progress—or if you think that the relationship isn't salvageable—it might be time to consider changing your doctor.

When to Break Up with Your Doctor

Are you wondering if it may be time to break things off with your doctor? There are a few red flags that should tip you off:

- Do they cut you off while you're talking about your problems?

- Do they never get back to you with your lab results so you're always left wondering?

- Are they failing to make eye contact to show that they're paying attention when you speak?

- Are you just not being heard?

These are all sure signs that it might be time to move on. But not every warning sign is necessarily a deal-breaker. I'll have patients who tell me that their cardiologist isn't working out, for example. They'll say that she has a terrible bedside manner, but they've been seeing her for five years, and they don't feel like switching doctors. And I'll ask, "Well, have you discussed this with her?" No. And I get it. That's a potentially awkward conversation to have. But here's what I recommend: If you think that there's anything in your relationship that's salvageable, then try to work at it. Tell your doctor something like, "I love coming here, but I just feel so rushed all the time." That one statement can make a huge difference. I promise you, if you tell your doctor that you feel like they're not giving you enough time or really listening when you speak, they'll make an effort the next time they see you.

So don't throw in the towel until you've worked on your relationship and given it a shot. And if it *still* doesn't improve? Well, then it's time to cut your losses and find someone better.

There are a few flat-out deal-breakers in my book, though:

- Is your doctor belittling you or dismissing your complaints?
- Do they demean you and make you feel like you're not intelligent enough to grasp certain concepts?
- Do they speak down to you?

If you answered yes to any of these questions, I encourage you to find a new doctor as soon as possible.

How to Break Up with Your Doctor

The purpose of this book is to hopefully figure out where you and your doctor are disconnected and take steps to fix that. But some patient-doctor relationships may be beyond salvageable, and that's okay to admit. So, if you've realized that your doctor isn't right for you, how do you break the news? You might be tempted to "ghost" them (that is, just stop seeing them without any explanation), but you owe it to them and their future patients to be honest and forthcoming with constructive feedback. First, express that you've had certain expectations that weren't met. Keep in mind that at this stage, you may receive an explanation or you may realize that there's been some miscommunication. Also, it's important to note that no matter how uncomfortable this feels, it's best to do this in person if you already have an appointment scheduled or on the phone, rather than via written communication like email, which leaves open too much potential for vagueness or continuing a pattern of miscommunication. But, if you're not comfortable with that, you can just leave and never come back, without an explanation, as many patients often do.

Finding a New Doctor

When you're looking for a new doctor, make sure to keep in mind what you did and didn't like about your relationship with your former doctor. Ask for recommendations from friends and family in your community. Ask them what they like about their doctor and maybe even what they don't like. If someone says their doctor is really nice and that's important to you, make a note of that. If another says their doctor helps them avoid medication for a certain ailment, and you like that approach, note that, too. Keep a list, and then see if the doctor you might be interested in seeing is taking new patients, is on your insurance plan, and has an opening for you.

At your first appointment with your new doctor, check to see if they hit the marks of what's important to you. Notice how they treat their staff, as this tells a lot about a person. If you feel comfortable, you can let your new doctor know what was missing in your former patient-doctor relationship. Take the bull by the horns and say, "I have some expectations. This is what I'm looking for." Having this type of open dialogue (remember, communication is one of the cornerstones) will help ensure that your relationship with your new doctor works out.

Don't give up on this new doctor after your first appointment though. Yes, during that first meeting you can draw upon feelings in your heart and gut, but sometimes it takes a couple of visits to really get warmed up. Your new doctor may also be a little reserved around a new patient, so keep that in mind, too. Give them a chance.

◀ BEHIND THE CURTAIN ▶

I once had a patient with hepatitis C, who had chronic back pain and needed to see a pain management specialist. Unfortunately, there weren't any in the city, so he came in to see me. This patient wanted opioids, insisting that the only thing that worked was taking five Vicodin each day. I told him that I didn't feel comfortable jumping straight to that prescription without first looking at options like physical therapy. He wasn't happy with that response. "You don't believe me," he told me. "You think I'm a drug addict. You don't know the level of my pain."

I didn't think he was a drug addict, but he was right about one thing: I didn't know the pain he was feeling. When a patient tells me they're in pain, I have to respect that. And that's exactly what I told him. But I also told him that the last thing either of us wanted to do was add on another problem of addiction.

He said, "No, doc, you don't have to worry about that. You don't understand. I chew them up like candy because my pain is so bad."

Still, I held fast to my belief. I had a responsibility to do what I thought was best for my patients and to do no harm. "I'm sorry that this visit isn't going the way you want it to go," I said. "But I can't in good conscience do this if we have other alternatives that I think are safer for you."

His reply? "Fine. I don't need you as my doctor. This isn't going to work. I'm not coming back here because you're not trying to help me."

As hard as that was to hear, I knew that he was actually right. It wasn't going to work out. We weren't a fit. No doctor can be the right doctor for *every* patient out there. And on this healthcare journey, that's what we're searching for: the right doctor-patient match.

From Doctor to Doctor

None of us wants an unhappy patient. While their unhappiness may have absolutely nothing to do with us and we can take steps to try to ease their pain, sometimes it may very well have to do with the fact that they simply don't resonate with us. When I have a patient I just can't develop a bond with, I have found these approaches helpful and maybe you will, too.

- I try not to take it personally if a patient discontinues their relationship with me. I realize that sometimes a patient and I are just not a match. I might ask what went wrong for my own knowledge, but once a patient has requested their records be sent to another doctor, there is nothing I can do to change their mind, and I wouldn't want to. I want to be able to give my attention to patients who want to be in my office and want me to be their doctor.

- Doctors can't "break up" with a patient the same way a patient can "break up" with us due to healthcare laws and regulations, but when I feel that a patient and I are having difficulty connecting, I will be very honest with them and say, "I don't think this relationship is working out for us. We're having some challenges as far as communication is concerned." If I have had a lot of interactions with a certain patient and no matter what I do we can't get on the same page and the relationship becomes a little argumentative or cynical, it is best for me to accept that the patient-doctor bond is going to be difficult to attain and be okay with that.

- If a patient expresses that they are unhappy with me and says something like "You know, you didn't listen to me last time" or "I wish you would have given me more time" or "You rushed me out of the office," I don't brush off their complaints by trying to defend myself. Criticism isn't easy to take, especially if we feel like we did the best we can, but if a patient is bringing something to my attention, I have to listen. When I listen, I might understand how the patient perceived something a certain way or I might be able to pick out some things I would like to change. If one patient brings something to my attention, I consider that maybe other patients are feeling the same way.

- Honestly, some patients are just not pleasant people and we might have no idea why. If a patient has a persistently negative attitude toward me, I will have that difficult discussion where I say something like, "Hey, look, what do you think about our interactions? For me, it feels like we are having a disconnect. I'm trying my best to work for you, but maybe you don't see it the same way. Maybe you are perceiving that I'm not giving you what you need. I don't want you to be in that position because your visit with me or with any doctor is supposed to be one where you feel like you're with a trusted member of your family." If we still can't get on the same page, I'll suggest that there are a lot of great physicians out there who may be better suited for them, and if I personally know that a certain doctor might be more their style, I won't hesitate to mention it. I am very careful about this conversation because I don't want the patient to think that I'm "breaking up" with them, but I do want them to know that I'm truly thinking of what might make them happier with their healthcare.

CHAPTER 7

A Conversation with Dr. Redcross:
Common Patient Questions Answered

Communication is one of the cornerstones of the patient-doctor bond. Now, I know that my conversation with you throughout this book has been a one-sided conversation, but I'm feeling pretty close to you because you now know a lot about me and how passionate I am about strengthening the patient-doctor bond. I want to close this book by answering some of the questions that several of my patients have asked me over the years that you might also have and maybe want to bring up with your own doctor at your next visit. These are brief answers. I could probably talk all day about some of them, so this isn't the be-all and end-all of the discussion. My answers are simply intended to help you get the conversation started.

Do you think natural medicines are an effective approach to healthcare?

I believe there is space for natural remedies and medicines to make a huge impact on healthcare. Yes, I am a Western-trained physician from Columbia Presbyterian and I still "bleed Columbia blue," but if there's one thing I've learned in my career—and over the course of my life—it's that some natural medicines and remedies do have some efficacy and good data supporting them. Certain natural medicines can even be quite effective. I've found myself researching these alternatives more and more often because some health complaints and conditions just don't require my prescription pad (which is my goal!). My patients appreciate that approach because they want to avoid the potential side effects of prescription medication whenever possible. I don't believe that natural medicine is a substitute for all Western medicine, but it is a good complement.

Do you believe that homeopathic remedies work?

Homeopathic remedies contain minute doses of natural substances, doses so small that some might conclude there is no way they could cause a significant effect on the body. They can be quite controversial because we don't have the typical Western placebo-controlled randomized studies backing them. With that said, some homeopathic remedies, such as arnica, are actually becoming more mainstream, and I do believe they can promote healing in certain cases. It is important to get homeopathic products from a reputable company, such as Boiron. A leader in homeopathy, Boiron has two homeopathic products that I wouldn't hesitate to suggest to my patients if the need was there: one is Arnicacare, which comes in a few different forms; it is used for bruising, pain, and swelling. The other is Oscilloccinum, which helps relieve symptoms associated with the flu. Keep in mind that even though homeopathy has the potential to make a big difference in our health, if you are not feeling better within a reasonable time, be sure to check with a homeopath and your medical doctor for further evaluation.

What do you think of Eastern medicine?

Ayurvedic medicine, traditional Chinese medicine, and other Eastern healing practices have been around for ages, and I totally respect them. I know they have helped a lot of people throughout the ages. I don't use those approaches in my practice (although I personally love acupuncture), but if a patient is interested in trying one of the healing practices associated with those approaches, I will spend my time researching what they are considering, and as long as I conclude it won't impede their healing, I'm all for it.

What do you think of Western medicine?

I'm Western trained; that's my base. I love being a physician, and I feel fortunate and blessed to be able to positively touch people's lives every day with the tools of modern medicine. Western medicine is science-based, and scientists are discovering new and better ways of healing on a daily basis. It's only going to get better as far as eliminating disease states and providing more options than we had in the past. In the not too distant future, medicine will become more personalized. Imagine going to the doctor, and from a simple blood test, the doctor will be able to prescribe a medicine that is designed solely for *you*! For Western medicine, the sky's the limit. I'm looking forward to seeing big-time cures for cancer and other disease states in the future thanks to the medical scientists who are researching around the clock to make that happen.

Can meditation and mindfulness practices help keep us healthy?

When I'm out on the road or on the radio, you'll hear me say that meditation and mindfulness are the number-one practices for staying healthy and happy. These practices are so essential to our health and well-being, but we often leave them out of our day, and maybe even our life. Sometimes we think that a pill or something tangible is the only thing that will make a difference, but that's just not true. There are many studies showing the importance of meditation for relieving anxiety, stress, and depression, which can lead to better overall health.

The idea of meditation scares some people off, but meditation can be as simple as three to four minutes of disconnecting from the world and listening to your breathing, of just being there for yourself. Each of us owes it to ourselves to be there for ourselves for at least a few minutes a day. Being present to ourselves in the moment with whatever is going on is mindfulness, whether that's during meditation or while opening the day's mail.

There's no one-size-fits-all way to unplug from the world. For me, that's meditation and mindfulness. For others, that might be tai chi, qi gong, prayer, dancing, mantra chanting, etc. Whatever it is, each of us should have a personal tool that we can call upon when we are having a rough time or just to get to that place where we feel refreshed.

What role does spirituality play in healthcare?

My approach to life and to my practice is spiritual. I believe in a source. Many of my patients do as well, whether that be Buddha, Jesus, Allah, the Universe, God, Higher Power, and so on. I'm not afraid to discuss spirituality with my patients. Regardless of one's religion, we are all just trying to get to that same place—that place of peace, happiness, and bliss. I can't say for other physicians what spirituality should mean to them in their practice, since spirituality is a very personal quality, but for me, it is my way to connect with my staff, my patients, with other doctors, and basically with whomever I come into contact with throughout the day.

Do you believe in the power of visualization?

I absolutely believe in the power of visualization to bring about positive changes in one's life, and I always recommend it to my patients. One of my favorite books on the topic is *Creative Visualization: Use the Power of Your Imagination to Create What You Want in Your Life* by Shakti Gawain. This book is a beautiful source for introducing visualization and meditation into your life.

I have a fun story with regard to visualization that really drove home for me how powerful the technique can be. So, like many others, I have always admired Oprah Winfrey and the journey she went on to achieve her success. I had always wanted to create a career that would allow me to marry medicine and media to touch more people, and I felt Oprah had skillfully married her own passion for changing lives with a highly successful media career. I wanted to emulate her success in my own practice. So, when I created a vision board to inspire and motivate myself, I included a photo of Oprah because I felt visualizing the level of success she had as being attainable in my own life would help me reach my goals. On that board, I also included the logos of some health networks I knew I wanted to do business with, as well as some television networks I admired and wanted to work with in order to reach more people and change more lives.

I looked at that vision board every day while I was growing my practice. That visual representation of the future I wanted helped me stay focused on my goal and create the outcome I wanted. Then, about eleven years later, I attended an awards ceremony with a friend in the entertainment industry. As I walked around, I bumped into someone. I looked up, and lo and behold, I'd literally bumped into Miss Oprah Winfrey herself! You can imagine how astonished I was because all I could do was look at her and say, "Hi, Miss Winfrey! How are you? You know, it's like we've met before."

She laughed and said, "Oh really now?"

Then she graciously obliged to take a picture with me. I truly believe my visualizing the life and career I wanted brought me to that serendipitous meeting. So, my answer is a resounding yes. I believe the power of willing your way to your goals and aspirations can have a genuine, tangible impact on where you go and what you accomplish in life. I want everybody to meet their Oprah Winfrey, whatever that may mean to them and to their heart, and I honestly think visualization can become a powerful tool for bringing oneself there, and that includes better health.

What sort of physical activity is best?

The type of physical activity that's right for someone depends on that person's age, condition, their preferences, and more. I personally love cross training and weight training; I like the feeling of soreness in my muscles after a grueling weight-training session, but I know there are plenty of people who aren't into that. Some people like power walking, rowing, cycling, aerobics, swimming . . . there are so many different activities to choose from.

According to the U.S. government, 80 percent of Americans don't meet the national activity recommendation requirement for aerobic or muscle training, and 3 percent of us cram a recommended week's worth of exercise into one or two days ("weekend warriors"). Only about one in three adults get the recommended amount of exercise and about 25 to 35 percent of adults are inactive. Studies show that 75 minutes of vigorous activity or 150 minutes of moderate exercise per week, as is recommended by the World Health Organization (WHO),[25] can lower one's risk of death due to cardiovascular disease by 40 percent and risk of death due to cancer by 18 percent, among other benefits. So it's not a matter of what physical activity is best; it's a matter of doing our best to work a regular exercise routine into our lives.

A good rule of thumb is to avoid doing too much too soon. Be patient, and make sure that you get some professional instruction at the gym, particularly with weight training, so you avoid overexertion or injury. Hurting yourself will only set you back further in your fitness goals, so take your time and make sure you're exercising safely. Also, make sure you're diversifying your activities as well, rather than just doing the same exercise every day, so your whole body can feel the benefits.

Warm up before you work out, and give yourself enough time to cool down after or between exercises. This will help you avoid injury.

Make sure you give any pain, swelling, or bruising the appropriate care, and that you don't "power through" any injury rather than making sure you've had time to heal. I personally use Arnicare, which is a homeopathic remedy for pain, to manage my exercise-related discomfort, and I highly recommend it. Some restorative foods, such as blueberries, can help with muscle soreness, too. Eggs are rich in amino acids, salmon is packed with omega-3 fatty acids, and ginger is anti-inflammatory and contains antioxidants—all of which help your body recover after exercise. Of course, hydration is essential to a well-rounded exercise regimen so make sure you're drinking enough water.

If you are considering starting an exercise program, by all means, speak with your doctor to discover what might be best for you.

How much sleep am I supposed to be getting?

Adults generally need at least seven hours of sleep a night. The CDC says adults should get at least seven hour of sleep a night. It is important not to skimp on this because sleep is an active process. During sleep, our body refreshes, repairs, and rejuvenates itself and keeps our immune system in good working order. Before I discuss this with them, not many of my patients realize how intimately related our immune system is to our quality of sleep. It takes only one sleepless night to throw off our immune system.

So when we talk about sleep, we need to talk about eliminating things that can keep us from getting a full night's rest:

alcohol, caffeine, and nicotine should all be avoided before bedtime and perhaps even several hours before bedtime. We also need to talk about things that can help us sleep better: some examples include tryptophan-rich walnuts, chamomile tea, magnesium-rich almonds, fish oil, and tart cherries (which contain melatonin, the "sleep hormone"). We also need to talk about other factors that can promote a restful sleep like a good pillow, mattress, blankets, bedsheets, and a cool room temperature.

And, if we're still not sleeping great for whatever reason, it is especially important to boost our immune system some other way: AHCC is a medicinal mushroom that is a powerful immune system booster, which I often recommend to patients. (See also "What are some steps I can take to boost my immune system?" on page 122.)

What's the best weight-loss regimen?

I might sound like a broken record when I say this, but the best weight-loss regimen is good old-fashioned watching your diet and exercising. Your body is a machine; you give it fuel and, if you want to lose weight, you burn more fuel than you take in. Now, when I say burn more fuel than we take in, we want to remember that the fuel we put in there needs to be clean fuel. We also want to support our body with enough water and fiber.

There's no quick fix or magic pill that will give you long-lasting weight loss. That's why your mental state is so important when it comes to weight loss. If you want to fit in that dress before your reunion and are willing to do anything you can to lose 10 pounds in two weeks, sure you'll look great in that dress, but two weeks later, it probably won't fit anymore.

This is why it is important to remember that our body does not define us; our spirit does. Or bodies are the outer shells of who we are, and inside we are spirit. We are more successful when we lose weight because we want our body to be a healthy home for our spirit rather than something to display to our old high school friends.

I'm not a big proponent for pills. Nor am I a big fan of weight-loss surgery except in cases where the patient's life would be at risk from the excess weight. Otherwise, diet and exercise is the way to go.

Should I be taking apple cider vinegar?

I hear this question so often that I've started to really take a look at the benefits of apple cider vinegar. I've seen lists and reports of all the suggested benefits, like support with diabetes management due to regulating blood sugar levels, weight loss, acne, gut health, and so on. These all sound really promising, so if you ask *should* you take it, my answer is, "If you'd like to try it, I support you. But let's make sure you are balancing it with everything else and that you're not overdoing it." Remember, although many natural remedies and a proper diet can support good health, no natural remedy or food is a replacement for traditional medicine.

What are some steps I can take to boost my immune system?

Number one is getting enough sleep (see page 120). Otherwise, there are a lot of really great foods and supplements that can give your immune system an edge, especially during cold and flu season. Some of these include AHCC, turmeric, onions, garlic, ginger, rosemary, raw honey, elderberry, fennel oil, echinacea, good old-fashioned chicken soup, bone broth, and homeopathic Oscilloccinum. Specifically with regard to AHCC, this medicinal mushroom is used in over 700 clinics throughout Asia. It's backed by many human clinical studies from several credible research institutions and has been shown to help fight infections and abnormal cell growth and boost immunity.[26] Ordinary mushrooms and other mushroom supplements I've looked into just don't have the powerful immune-stimulating action that AHCC does, so it is definitely one of my preferred immune boosters. I could go on about the benefits of the other foods and supplements I mentioned, but that could take a whole book. The idea I really want to impart here is that there is an arsenal of healthy foods and supplements at your disposal to boost your immune system.

Should I take a multivitamin/mineral? What other supplements should I take?

A long time ago, our foods were rich in all the vitamins and minerals we needed. Unfortunately, our soil has been pretty much depleted of these essential nutrients and so our plant foods do not have the same levels of vitamins and minerals they once had.[27] Also, our nutritional demands have increased because our bodies are constantly combatting environmental toxins and stress. So, yes, I recommend taking quality vitamins and minerals. There are many other supplements on the market as well. For example, most cardiologists will recommend that their patients take fish oil capsules and coenzyme Q10, and gastroenterologists often recommend a probiotic supplement to their patients to support gut health because so much of our immune system is housed in the lining of our gut.

One vitamin I'm really passionate about is vitamin D. Vitamin D is currently the third most common vitamin deficiency in America, which is alarming because vitamin D has an important role in our health on so many levels. For one, it is essential to the health of our immune system and it may even affect our sense of well-being. Low levels of vitamin D have been implicated in a variety of chronic disease states, including obesity. According to a 2008 study, vitamin D deficiency is linked to health risks in thirty-six target organs in the body and can increase one's risk of diseases like osteoporosis, heart disease, and cancer.[28] Another study published in 2010 indicates that insufficient levels of vitamin D can negatively impact over 200 genes in the human body.[29] These studies and others like them strongly suggest that vitamin D is one of the vitamins we should be taking daily.

You might wonder, "But don't we get vitamin D from the sun?" That's true, but our skin (with half the body exposed) needs twenty minutes of exposure to sunlight without burning to produce vitamin D; these days, not many people venture out into the sun without being covered from head to toe in sun protection—and for good reason: The sun can be dangerous. Moreover, people who have more melanin in their skin (for example, African Americans and Latinos) may not produce enough vitamin D in those twenty minutes and would need to stay out longer, but that's often not feasible. Others at risk for vitamin D deficiency include office workers (due to the lack of sunlight) and adults over age fifty-five because the skin of an aging body is generally less efficient at synthesizing vitamin D.[30]

This is why it's so necessary for us to make sure that we are getting vitamin D in our diet, which can be a real challenge, especially for vegans and vegetarians. So, what do we do? Supplement with this and other essential and nonessential nutrients and have our blood tested with your doctor to ensure we're getting adequate amounts of vitamin D. (You can also order an at-home vitamin D test kit online from www.nutrient power.org.)

We're having difficulty getting pregnant; are there any natural approaches we can try to support our efforts?

Millions of people are affected by infertility for various medical reasons, so I answer this question only after medical problems have been ruled out and a couple is still having difficulty conceiving. For starters, is the couple being intimate often enough? You would be surprised that this is often the cause of a failure to get pregnant. When trying to get pregnant, frequency during ovulation is very important. We also need to consider factors such as environmental toxins, poor diet, immune challenges, poor lifestyle choices, obesity, high levels of stress, alcohol consumption, and smoking. All, some, or even one of these things may be affecting a couple's ability to get pregnant.

When trying to get pregnant, it's advisable for women to eat fewer meat-based proteins, more plant source proteins like nuts, more whole grains with fiber and vitamin E and B, more fruits and vegetables, and less dairy and caffeine. Prenatal vitamins are hugely important for women who are looking to get pregnant, especially vitamins E, A, D, B, and folic acid. For men, a 1996 study illustrates that an increase in L-carnitine in the body directly parallels an increase in sperm motility,[31] so taking L-carnitine supplements can help improve the health of the sperm, thereby increasing the chances of pregnancy. Always avoid hazardous environmental toxins, including BPAs, phthalates in makeup and plastic, high amounts of fluoride, and MSG.

I don't mean to say that any of this is a replacement for medical intervention if necessary. What I'm suggesting is that there are natural ways to help support fertility and encourage pregnancy in couples who don't have additional medically based fertility issues. There are several good books on the topic of how to improve your chances of conceiving naturally, and I encourage anyone with this concern to read as much as they can and follow the recommendations that seem right for them, in addition to speaking with their OBGYN.

How can I avoid a stroke?

Strokes are a leading cause of disability in America, so it is something we *all* want to take steps to avoid. About 12 million strokes occur every year, and many are preventable. A stroke is a "brain attack," and there are four types to be familiar with: 1) Ischemic stroke, which account for nine out of ten strokes. This is a case of not getting enough blood to the brain. 2) Hemorrhagic stroke is where a blood vessel ruptures in the brain. 3) Transient ischemic attack (TIA) is a "mini stroke" in which blood flood is temporarily blocked to the brain. 4) Silent stroke does not present with any symptoms but causes damage in the brain.

Staying on top of your blood pressure is one of the most important things you can do to protect yourself from a stroke. You can even get a blood pressure cuff that syncs to your smartphone, making it really easy to keep tabs on it. Taking action to rectify sleep apnea and reducing high cholesterol are two more important steps. Another good approach is to eat brain-healthy foods like garlic, caffeine (yes, in moderation), olive oil, sweet potatoes, fruits, vegetables, and egg yolks.

Citicholine is a naturally occurring brain chemical, which decreases as we get older. It's available in supplement form and has been shown to protect the fats in the cell membranes, especially in our brains. In over 100 human clinical trials, it has been shown to aid in brain cell recovery. Within four hours following a stroke, citicholine has been found to repair damage.[32]

I sometimes google my symptoms. Do you have a website that you think is a reputable one to check? And what do you think about those sites that let you chat with a live doctor?

WebMD and Medscape are good choices, but don't rely on them without speaking to your doctor. As far as chatting with a doctor you have never met over the internet, I have to say that I don't really think that's a great idea. You are missing out on so much, and for a doctor to really have a good idea of what's going on for you at all levels, they need to physically be in the room with you. This whole book is about the patient-doctor bond, and this just isn't possible with an impersonal online visit. We are people, and we need to exchange energy. Let's always remember that there's a bigger source than all of us out there, and it isn't the worldwide web. We need to come together to heal and thrive.

How often do I really need to see my doctor?

You should see your doctor at least once a year for your annual exam. I even like a six-month check-in because a lot can happen in a year. Of course if you have specific healthcare needs, you'll need to see your doctor more frequently.

Can mental stress really cause physical illness?

Absolutely! Back when I first worked in Los Angeles, I was also a part owner of a small urgent care facility in Sacramento, over an hour away by plane. I had a business partner who ran the clinic, and I would fly in every week in my role as president of the organization to make sure everything was running smoothly because the day-to-day goings-on of the clinic were my responsibility. As you can imagine, I began to experience a great deal of stress. I stopped taking adequate care of myself; I didn't get enough sleep, and I didn't eat as well as I normally would.

This stress piled up until one day, on my way to catch my weekly flight, I took myself to the emergency room at the hospital where I worked in Los Angeles, thinking I was coming down with an upper respiratory infection because my chest felt heavy, and I couldn't tolerate my normal exercise regimen. I underwent blood tests, chest x-rays, and several EKGs. The EKGs read that I was experiencing an acute myocardial infarction, or a heart attack. I then underwent cardiac catherization, which revealed that my coronary arteries were open, which later confirmed that I had Takotsubo syndrome. This is a stress-induced condition that affects healthy young adults that, luckily, is reversible for most—but not without a lot of work. I spent a month confined to my home recovering from the syndrome that resulted in heart failure, taking several medications to protect and heal my damaged heart. The side effects were worse for me than the disease itself.

This event rearranged the priorities in my life. It shifted my perspective outward to focus on how the amount of stress in my life impacted the lives of my patients. If I'd just gotten on the plane that day, I might not have walked off it. I don't allow stress to run my life anymore, and I strive to help my patients keep stress from running theirs. My own near-death changed the way I viewed not only the patient-doctor bond but also the way I approach the seriousness of stress and its influence over our health.

If you could only offer your patients one piece of advice, what would that be?

I truly believe that being in optimal health boils down to these three essential principles: 1) good nutrition, 2) regularly moving our bodies, and 3) believing in something greater than ourselves (spirituality, that is). Our early ancestors had it right: Physical movement was required for hunting and gathering, and just about anything else they needed to do. The food they ate was freshly killed or picked and packed full of all the nutrients a body needs. They also had deep spiritual beliefs as evidenced by the cave paintings they left behind. Remember, spirituality and religion aren't necessarily synonymous, so I'm not suggesting that my patients suddenly take up a religious practice. When I talk about spirituality, I'm talking about believing in yourself, believing in opportunities, believing in the universe—whatever you may call it—to really give yourself a fighting chance in life.

Let's say 'em together: Nutrition, Movement, and Spirituality. Get these three things in order and your chances of being the healthiest you can be increases a thousandfold.

Doc, how do you keep yourself healthy?

I do my best to practice what I preach. I try to make sure that not only am I doing what I need to do to stay physically and mentally healthy but also spiritually healthy. For me, my spirituality is around meditation and visualization, where I can check in with myself to make sure that I am in alignment with my values and create the life that I want to lead. I'm not perfect; I'm a work in progress, and I work at it each and every day. I'm just like the patients I sit with on a daily basis: far from perfect but doing my best.

Conclusion

Thank you for taking the time to read about my passion to help you achieve "patient nirvana" and increase healthcare happiness across the country. I believe it is a blessing to be able to impart some helpful information to you with regard to strengthening your relationship with your doctor. Hopefully, this information will allow you to create the bond with your doctor I know you deserve.

I feel so fortunate to be able to share so much of me and who I am with my patients, and I hope that you feel you're able to share much of who you are with your physician. I do know how challenging it can be to get on the same page as your doctor—and vice versa. There's so much standing in the way of developing a solid bond. In addition to all the roadblocks I discussed throughout this book, things like stress, physician burnout, health insurance hassles, unrealistic expectations, and more can block the way. So, while it does take effort, together we can push aside those roadblocks to make way for healthier relationships in medicine.

I look forward to a future where more people achieve "patient nirvana" because developing trust, communication, respect, and empathy in the patient-doctor relationship is made a priority at each and every visit. With these four cornerstones in place, you and your doctor can have positive interactions, get to the root of any health problems quicker, and bring about your best possible health together.

I encourage you to share this book with your doctor or any doctors you might know as well as with your family members and friends. The more people who read this and make a sincere effort to make a strong patient-doctor bond a reality, the more I will have fulfilled my passion to change lives for the better. I couldn't ask for more. And for that, I thank you.

Author's Note
to Fellow Doctors

"You can't ever reach perfection, but you can believe in an asymptote toward which you are ceaselessly striving."

—Dr. Paul Kalanithi

Mrs. Berkowitz was a sweet and world-worn elderly woman, at the very least ninety years old. She was punctual, but she was also quite loquacious, which wasn't exactly convenient for me and my long day. I had been loaded with countless seemingly insurmountable tasks that would surely keep me in the office until the wee hours of the morning. Yet something prompted me to ask Mrs. Berkowitz a question that would quickly turn my day around and forever change our relationship. "Mrs. Berkowitz," I asked, sitting cross-legged at the foot of the stool upon which she perched, "will you tell me about what in your life has made you who you are?"

She began to speak about spending a portion of her life

133

in Europe, though not on vacation like I have. No, she told me that she spent time there against her will. I didn't catch on to her meaning at first. It wasn't until she slowly raised her shirtsleeve that I began to understand. Tattooed on her forearm were several numbers. She said that she had been to hell and back. She had been at Auschwitz. Mrs. Berkowitz had lived through imprisonment in a concentration camp, had lost her parents and siblings, and had seen unspeakable horrors. She was able to escape thanks to an angelic family, eventually finding freedom. And now, by some miracle, she was here with me, telling me about her most painful memories and trusting me with her care.

I can't tell you how thankful I was to meet Mrs. Berkowitz and to hear her story. There I was complaining about my workload, late nights, and how life wasn't fair. Let me tell you, that was the last time I ever felt sorry for myself. After listening to Mrs. Berkowitz, I realized that I wouldn't have had the strength to survive such an ordeal. I was honored to care for a real hero.

It's patients like Mrs. Berkowitz who remind me why I do what I do—what all doctors do. The description for what a physician does today dates back to the 1500s, but the first physician was believed to have been an Egyptian in 2600 B.C. We are in an old and noble profession, one in which we self-lessly serve in the interest of the people. We make a difference.

This is a beautiful truth that we've somehow forgotten.

According to a recent survey, eight out of ten physicians are "somewhat pessimistic or very pessimistic about the future of the medical profession."[33] In 1973, 85 percent of physicians had no doubts about their career choice, while in 2008, only 6 percent could describe their morale as positive. More distressing, today's doctors are feeling more down than ever before.

This isn't okay. And clearly something is missing. What is that something? It's a true and deep connection with patients on a human level that feeds our soul and allows us to feel that we are fulfilling our life's purpose.

If we want to fix healthcare, if we want to have happier and healthier patients and doctors, we must recommit ourselves to the patient-doctor bond. Of course, this commitment to building and maintaining a bond isn't so much a solution as it is an ongoing process.

It's not a solitary process. It takes patients and doctors working together and doing their part, each contributing to the relationship. It requires that we each realize where we've done wrong and then course-correcting. It takes pledging ourselves to each other, being in it together.

It's not a short process. It requires taking small steps over long periods of time. It requires patience. It requires forgiveness. And it requires trying again next time and the time after that.

It's not an easy process. It requires us giving so much of ourselves. It requires our vulnerability. It requires our effort. It's something that we have to think about, have to work at.

But let me tell you something: It's worth it. Ultimately, this isn't just about the healthiness of our bodies—it's about the happiness of our hearts, the nourishment of our souls.

It's about changing lives. And we all have the power—the responsibility—to do it.

Promise me you'll try.

THE REDCROSS PLEDGE
"To Change Lives"

I pledge to **educate, encourage, and inspire** you to become actively involved in your health and wellness.

I pledge to ensure you have a **pleasing and satisfying** visit.

I pledge, when treatment is necessary, to provide the **highest quality** care available anywhere in the medical community.

I pledge to provide you with a clear explanation and plan as to how I intend to keep you **healthy and whole.**

I pledge to have myself or one of my team members **available** when you need us.

I pledge to treat you **as I would also wish to be treated.**

NOW HELP ME HELP YOU

I take my responsibility to fulfill my pledge to you very seriously and building a long-term quality relationship with you is my highest goal. In order for me to fulfill my pledge to you, I need your help.

I ask you to strive for the following:

TO have a **positive attitude, open mind to learn, and be motivated** to become actively involved in preventing dis"ease."

TO know that no matter what you may be dealing with you are **healthy** in my mind and I want you to **feel** that way as well.

TO try and arrive on time for your appointment so that I can fully provide **you** with the time you deserve.

The Redcross Pledge

Acknowledgments

So where do I begin? I have so many people to thank for all of my blessings. Never would I have imagined that a project I started in 2007 would take "only" eleven years to complete! I am so happy to have finally poured my soul into this book with the hope that it will leave you happier than you were before you read it.

None of this would have been possible without the best family on Earth, starting with my wonderful and supportive wife, Natalie, and the world's best twins, Evan and Sophia! I love you guys for dealing with my early mornings and sleepless nights to make my dream a reality. Thank you, thank you, and thank you. I also thank my parents, William and Patricia Redcross, for instilling in me the values that taught me that if you're not working to improve the quality of someone else's life, what's the point? You're the two best friends an only child could ever ask for.

When you write something as personal as a book, you have so many people who are instrumental in helping you put things together, whether it be through organization or inspiration. I especially want to thank Dave Kerpen, Chairman of Likeable Media, for providing me with both. Thank you, Dave, for helping me to think "BIG" and making sure the process was "likeable" all the way through.

I gratefully acknowledge Judge Greg Mathis, who honored me with his kind and thoughtful words in the Foreword to this book.

I am also greatly appreciative to Carol Killman Rosenberg and her equally talented husband, Gary Rosenberg, for sharing their book publishing expertise with me throughout the process of getting my book ready for publication. Special thanks to Theresa Braun for her valuable assistance, as well.

I also want to thank the hospitals, practices, and my colleagues from the East Coast to the West Coast. Each of the stories I share in this book were born from my experiences and education along the way from some very special institutions and even more special fellow physicians (Dr. Dan Stone, Dr. Tina Koopersmith, Dr. Tom Price, Dr. Stacey Rosenbaum, Dr. Ilan Kedan, and many others), and I am so grateful. I also wanted to thank all of the nurses, phlebotomists, ward clerks, PAs, NPs, office managers, custodial engineers, and so many more, who showed me kindness and support along the way, allowing me to live out my purpose and learn to better foster a BOND with my patients. And a special thank-you to Mike Weaver, one of the producers of *The Doctors,* who planted the seed of writing this book.

There are many other people throughout my life who have also provided support and inspiration, but there are too many to name here. Please know that you have my utmost appreciation.

Last, but definitely not least, I thank all of you—not just those of you who believe in my message and were kind enough to read my book, but also all the patients who have entrusted me with their care and allowed me into their soul, while providing me with invaluable lessons on how to create a true BOND.

References

1 Association of American Medical Colleges. "New Research Confirms Looming Physician Shortage." AAMC. April 5, 2016. Last accessed February 20, 2017. www.aamc.org/newsroom/newsreleases/458074/2016 _workforce_projections_04052016.html.

2 Schwartz, MD, Mark D.; Steven Durning, MD; Mark Linzer, MD; et al. "Changes in Medical Students' Views of Internal Medicine Careers from 1990 to 2007." *Arch Intern Med.* 171(8) (2011): 744–749. doi:10.1001/archinternmed.2011.139.

3 Hamblin, James. "What Doctors Make: Variations in Salary Are Drastic and Opaque." The Atlantic. January 27, 2015. Last accessed February 20, 2018. www.theatlantic.com/health/archive/2015/01/physician-salaries /384846.

4 Cheung, PharmD, Kevin; Jacob Hicks, PharmD; Brian McEwen; and Gregory Cianfarani, RPh. "Strong Healthcare Provider-Patient Relationship Improves Patient Adherence and Lowers Healthcare Costs: A Meta-Analysis." Last accessed February 20, 2018. mycred.com/libs/pdf/healthcare_portfolios_patient_adherence.pdf.

5 Halpern, MD, PhD, Jodi. "What is Clinical Empathy?" *J Gen Intern Med* 18(8) (August 2003): 670–674. doi:10.1046/j.1525-1497.2003.21017.x.

6 Laurie, Esther. "Brene Brown's Definition of Trust Will Change Your Relationships." Church Leaders. December 30, 2015. Accessed March 29, 2018. churchleaders.com/daily-buzz/269819-brene-browns-definition-of-trust-will-change-your-relationships.html.

7 Bergland, Christopher. "How Does the Vagus Nerve Convey Instincts to the Brain?" *Psychology Today.* May 23, 2014. Accessed March 29, 2018. www.psychologytoday.com/blog/the-athletes-way/201405/how-does-the-vagus-nerve-convey-gut-instincts-the-brain.

8 Covey, Stephen. *The Speed of Trust: The One Thing That Changes Everything.* New York: Free Press, 2008.

9 Esposito, Lisa. "Health Buzz: Many Patients Lie to Their Doctors, Survey Finds." *U.S. News.* November 10, 2015. Accessed March 29, 2018. health.usnews.com/health-news/health-wellness/articles/2015/11/10/many-patients-lie-to-their-doctors-survey-finds.

10 Terry, P. E., and M. L. Healey. "The Physician's Role in Educating Patients. A Comparison of Mailed Versus Physician-Delivered Patient Education." *Journal of Family Practice* 49, no. 4 (April 2000):314–8. www.ncbi.nlm.nih.gov/pubmed/10778836.

11 Patterson, Kerry, Joseph Grenny, Ron McMillan, and Al Switzler. *Crucial Conversations: Tools for Talking When Stakes Are High.* 2nd Ed. New York; McGraw-Hill Education, 2011.

12 Fong Ha, MBBS (Hons), Jennifer; Dip Surg Anat; and Nancy Longnecker, PhD. "Doctor-Patient Communication: A Review." *The Ochsner Journal* 10, no. 1 (Spring 2010):38–43. www.ncbi.nlm.nih.gov/pmc/articles/PMC3096184/.

13 Travaline, MD, John M.; Robert Ruchinskas, PsyD; and Gilbert E. D'Alonzo Jr, DO. "Patient-Physician Communication: Why and How." *Journal of the American Osteopathic Association* 105 (January 2005): 13–18. jaoa.org/article.aspx?articleid=2093086.

14 Fong Ha, MBBS, Jennifer, and Nancy Longnecker, PhD. "Doctor-Patient Communication: A Review." *Ochsner Journal* 10(1) (2010): 38–43. www.ncbi.nlm.nih.gov/pmc/articles/PMC3096184.

15 Marvel, M. K., R. M. Epstein, K. Flowers, and H. B. Beckman. "Soliciting the Patient's Agenda: Have We Improved?" *JAMA* 281(3) (January 1999): 283–7. www.ncbi.nlm.nih.gov/pubmed/9918487?dopt=Abstract.

16 Kessels, PhD, Roy P. C. "Patients' Memory for Medical Information." *J R Soc Med* 96(5) (May 2003): 219–222. www.ncbi.nlm.nih.gov/pmc/articles/PMC539473.

References

17 Institute for Healthcare Improvement. "Ask Me 3: Good Questions for Your Good Health." Last accessed February 20, 2018. www.npsf .org/?page=askme3.

18 Taiwo, N. *The Top Ten Laws of Respect*. Maitland, FL: Xulon Press, 2009.

19 Dickert, N. W., and N. E. Kass. "Understanding Respect: Learning from Patients." *J Med Ethics* 35(7) (July 2009): 419–423. doi:10.1136/ jme.2008.027235.

20 Covey, Stephe*n. 7 Habits of Highly Effective People*. New York City, NY: Free Press, 2009.

21 O'Rourke, Meghan. "Doctors Tell All—and It's Bad." *The Atlantic*. November 2014. Last accessed February 20, 2018. www.theatlantic.com/ magazine/archive/2014/11/doctors-tell-all-and-its-bad/380785.

22 Syed, MD, MSc, Fatima Z. "Unhappily Employed." *Annals of Internal Medicine Fresh Look*. February 14, 2018. Accessed March 29, 2018. freshlook.annals.org/2018/02/unhappily-employed.html?m=1.

23 Kao, MD, Helen; Rebecca Conant, MD; Theresa Soriano, MD, MPH; and Wayne McCormick, MD, MPH. "The Past, Present, and Future of House Calls." *Clinics in Geriatric Medicine* 25, no. 1 (February 2009): 19–34. www.geriatric.theclinics.com/article/S0749-0690(08)00063-3/ fulltext.

24 Miller, Anna Medaris. "Is the House Call Doctor Coming Back?" *U.S. News*. April 14, 2015. Accessed March 26, 2018. health.usnews.com /health-news/patient-advice/articles/2015/04/14/is-the-house-call-doctor -coming-back.

25 World Health Organization. "Physical Activity: Fact Sheet." WHO.int. Accessed April 23, 2018. www.who.int/mediacentre/factsheets/fs385/en/.

26 AHCC Research Association. "What Is AHCC?" AHCCResearch.com. Accessed April 23, 2018. ahccresearch.com/index.html.

27 Valint, Simon. "Vitamin D and Obesity." *Nutrients* 5, no. 3 (March 2013): 949–956. doi:10.3390/nu5030949.

28 Norman, BA, MS, PhD, Anthony W. "From Vitamin D to Hormone D: Fundamentals of the Vitamin D Endocrine System Essential for Good

Health." *American Journal of Clinical Nutrition* 2, vol. 88 (August 2008): 491S–499S.

29 Ramagopalan, Sreeram V., Andreas Heger, Antonio J. Berlanga, Narelle J. Maugeri, Matthew R. Lincoln, Amy Burrell, Lahiru Handunnetthi, Adam J. Handel, et al. "A ChIP-Seq-Defined Genome-Wide Map of Vitamin D Receptor Binding: Associations with Disease and Evolution." *Genome Research* 20 (October 2010): 1352–1360. doi: 10.1101/gr.107920.110.

30 Boucher, Barbara J. "The Problems of Vitamin D Insufficiency in Older People." *Aging Dis* 3, no. 4 (August 2012): 313–329. www.ncbi.nlm.nih .gov/pmc/articles/PMC3501367/.

31 Jeulin, Claudette, and Lawrence M. Lewin. "Role of Free L-Carnitine and Acetyl-L-Carnitine in Post-Gonadal Maturation of Mammalian Spermatozoa." *Hum Reprod Update* 2, no. 2 (1996): 87–102. www.ncbi.nlm .nih.gov/pubmed/9079406.

32 Centers for Disease Control and Prevention. "Stroke Facts." CDC .gov. Accessed April 23, 2018. www.cdc.gov/stroke/facts.htm; Quanhe Yang, PhD1; Xin Tong, MPH1; Linda Schieb, MSPH1; Adam Vaughan, PhD1; Cathleen Gillespie, MS1; Jennifer L. Wiltz, MD1; Sallyann Coleman King, MD1, et al. "Vital Signs: Recent Trends in Stroke Death Rates—United States, 2000–2015." *MMWR Morb Mortal Wkly* 66, no. 35 (Rep September 2017): 933–939. www.cdc.gov/mmwr/volumes/66/wr/mm6635e1. htm.; Secades, MD, PhD, Julio J. "Citicoline: Pharmacological and Clinical Review." *Rev Neurol.* 23, no. 63(S03) (December 2016): S1–S73, www.researchgate.net/publication/317167480_Citicoline_pharmacological_and_clinical_review_2016_update.

33 O'Rourke, Meghan. "Doctors Tell All—and It's Bad." *The Atlantic*. November 2014. Last accessed February 20, 2018. www.theatlantic.com/ magazine/archive/2014/11/doctors-tell-all-and-its-bad/380785.

About the Author

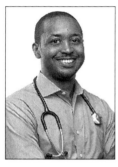 **Dr. Redcross** is a board-certified Internal Medicine physician. His expertise is capturing how to best provide the ultimate patient experience for those who may be concerned or frustrated with the deterioration of the patient-doctor relationship or for patients interested in developing or strengthening an existing relationship.

Dr. Redcross has worked with a diverse group of patients—from migrant farm workers, to the elderly, to patients battling drug addiction. His concierge approach has led to the development of an impressive following of patients from the entertainment industry, sports arena, and business world, spanning from Los Angeles to New York City.

Dr. Redcross has made several appearances on major media, including *The Doctors, Entertainment Tonight, The Insider,* CNN and HLN. He is frequently called on as an expert at media networks and syndicates across the country for his expertise in health and wellness.

In 2001, Dr. Redcross completed his medical training at the prestigious Columbia-Presbyterian Medical Center, followed by providing care in rural Oxnard, California. He then transitioned to the renowned Cedars-Sinai Medical Center in Beverly Hills, during which time he received the Man of Valor Award from the NAACP Youth Council for excellence in medicine. He created his Concierge practice in 2007 and established his company, Redcross Communications, Inc., under which he provides medical education through various media outlets including TV, radio, and print. His company, Redcross Wellness, creates elite, affordable nutritional supplements infused with nutrients that promote health and wellness.

Dr. Redcross participated in fellowships in Puerto Rico and the Dominican Republic, which contributed to his proficiency in Spanish. He embraces both natural and alternative methods of healing in his practice connecting spirituality, movement, and nutrition. Dr. Redcross's mission is to ensure that patients feel inspired, highly valued, and, above all, empowered.

Please visit Dr. Redcross online at www.drkenredcross.com.